SPIRITUALITY AND CHILDBIRTH

Highlighting aspects of birth often taken for granted, ignored or left silenced, this book questions the art and meaning of childbirth. Addressing spirituality in and around the start of life from a variety of thought-provoking perspectives, it examines the apparent paradox of impersonal biomedical-technocratic systems operating alongside the meaningful experiences encountered by those involved. Themes covered include:

- Notions of holism and spirituality, culture, religion and spirituality
- Childbirth significance at societal level
- Spiritual care in maternity care provision
- Birth environment, mood, space and place
- Spiritual experience of all those involved, including health professionals
- Spiritual experience when birth is complex and challenging
- When birth and death are juxtaposed.

Although there is considerable literature on spirituality at the end of life, this is the only book that draws together a global and multidisciplinary selection of academic researchers and practitioners to reflect on spirituality at the start of life. Each chapter explores the relevant theoretical background and makes links to practice, using case studies from research and practice. The chapters conclude by discussing: how spiritual care is, and should be, provided in this context; what practice approaches are beneficial; cross-cultural perspectives; and future directions for research. It is an important read for all those interested in childbirth, maternity care, social science perspectives on health and illness, and spirituality.

Susan Crowther is Professor of Midwifery at Robert Gordon University, UK.

Jenny Hall is Senior Lecturer in Midwifery at Bournemouth University, UK.

SPIRITUALITY AND CHILDBIRTH

Meaning and Care at the Start of Life

Edited by Susan Crowther and Jenny Hall

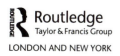

Routledge
Taylor & Francis Group

LONDON AND NEW YORK

First published 2018
by Routledge
2 Park Square, Milton Park, Abingdon, Oxon OX14 4RN

and by Routledge
711 Third Avenue, New York, NY 10017

Routledge is an imprint of the Taylor & Francis Group, an informa business

British Library Cataloguing-in-Publication Data
A catalogue record for this book is available from the British Library

Library of Congress Cataloging-in-Publication Data
Names: Crowther, Susan (Professor of midwifery), editor. | Hall, Jenny (Lecturer in midwifery), editor.
Title: Spirituality and childbirth : meaning and care at the start of life / edited by Susan Crowther and Jenny Hall.
Description: New York, NY : Routledge, [2017] | Includes bibliographical references and index.
Identifiers: LCCN 2017022428| ISBN 9781138229402 (hardback) | ISBN 9781138229419 (pbk.) | ISBN 9781315389646 (ebook)
Subjects: | MESH: Parturition--psychology | Pregnancy--psychology | Spirituality | Mother-Child Relations--psychology | Infant Care--psychology
Classification: LCC RG652 | NLM WQ 300 | DDC 618.4--dc23
LC record available at https://lccn.loc.gov/2017022428

ISBN: 978-1-138-22940-2 (hbk)
ISBN: 978-1-138-22941-9 (pbk)
ISBN: 978-1-315-38964-6 (ebk)

Typeset in Bembo
by HWA Text and Data Management, London

CONTENTS

FIGURES AND TABLES

Figures

Tables

CONTRIBUTORS

Alison Barrett, Canadian-trained specialist OBGYN and maternal and physician health advocate, currently working as a consultant obstetrician and gynaecologist in Aotearoa, New Zealand. Alison serves on the professional advisory group for La Leche League New Zealand, as well as actively supporting mothers in the community as a La Leche League group leader. Alison is a founding member of a popular social media-based support group for women doctors that seek to address the particular challenges and inequities that New Zealand women in medicine face. Alison is a member of OraTaia, the New Zealand Climate and Health Council, and is a trustee for the Home Birth Aotearoa Trust.

Sílvia Caldeira, Invited Assistant Professor of Nursing at Universidade Católica Portuguesa, Lisbon, Portugal. Sílvia's work focuses on spirituality in health, particularly in nursing care. Her master's in Bioethics (2008) relates to the ethical imperative of the inclusion of spirituality in nursing care, and her PhD (2013) covered the validation of nursing diagnosis spiritual distress from NANDA International. Sílvia published a book in Portuguese about spirituality in nursing (2011) and has published several papers and communications about this subject. She is an elected member of the Diagnosis Development Committee of NANDA International; coordinator of the NANDA-I Portugal Network Group; member of the Centre for Spirituality Studies, University of Hull (UK); member of the European Spirituality Nursing and Midwifery Research Network; member of the International Association for Spiritual Care; and member of the Global Network for Spirituality and Health.

Susan Crowther, Registered midwife. Professor of Midwifery at Robert Gordon University Aberdeen, Scotland. Susan has practised as a midwife in many countries in various roles, e.g. caseload midwife (urban and rural regions), group practice midwife and educator, an aid worker in low-income settings, consultant midwife and researcher. Her PhD was on the experience of being at birth and was titled 'Sacred Joy at Birth'. Susan currently leads on maternal, family and child wellbeing research. She regularly writes book chapters, peer-reviewed articles, and is on the editorial boards of four journals and reviews for others. She is a member of the International Confederation of Midwives' (ICM) Research Standing Committee (RSC). Susan's professional interests are myriad, the main ones being: continuity of carer within maternity, professional role of the midwife, sustainable practice, spirituality and childbirth, rural and remote maternity services and hermeneutic phenomenology. The overarching theme of Susan's work is relationality. Blog: drsusancrowther.com and Twitter: @susancrowtherMW

José Miguel de Angulo has more than 20 years' experience in community-focused public health practices for underserved populations around the world. José earned his medical degree in 1978 from the Universidad del Cauca in Colombia. He then pursued a Master of Public Health degree from the Johns Hopkins University in Baltimore, USA, in 1985. He joined MAP International in 1986 and, since 2009, has been the Latin America Regional Director for MAP International. He and his wife have been working within Community Health Programs with an emphasis on maternal and childcare, particularly comprehensive early infancy development and child protection. They have co-authored over 20 books and developed many educational materials on education, health determinants, holistic development, women and children's human rights, comprehensive early infancy development from a neuro-psycho-sociological perspective, and sexual violence against children.

Jenny Hall, Senior Midwifery Lecturer and researcher, Bournemouth University. Jenny has been in involved in midwifery for more than 30 years along with educating in some capacity all this time. Her passion is to view families holistically, including recognising spirituality, and she has published widely on these topics. Her doctoral holistic project explored the meaning of being a midwife and the art of midwifery practice, using creative methods including a reflective textile quilt. Recent completed research includes educating for promoting dignity and respect, the experiences of disabled women, and linking spirituality and infertility. She loves student midwives and telling stories about the 'old days'. She leads a unit on the Postgraduate Certificate for Education, developing educators. She recently became Senior Fellow of the Higher Education Authority. Jenny has a patient husband and five daughters, all born at home, who have no intention of being midwives – yet. Follow her on twitter @hallmum5

Carolyn Hastie, Mother, grandmother and midwife with qualifications in adult education, counselling, lactation, primary health care, reproductive and sexual health, New South Wales, New Zealand. Carolyn has been at the leading edge of midwifery practice and education for four decades. Now a freelance consultant midwife, having wide-ranging national and international experience in diverse settings, her work, including commissioning and managing a quality award-winning stand-alone midwifery service in New South Wales, is well known. Her passion is strengthening midwifery and improving care for childbearing women, partners and babies; her focus is on the neurophysiological intersection of growth, development and relationships. Areas of interest include neuroscience, epigenetics, the Polyvagal Theory, Barker's Theory, teamwork, social, emotional and spiritual intelligence, labour, birth, breastfeeding and attachment. She has researched, taught and written extensively on midwifery-related subjects. A core aspect of Carolyn's work is finding ways to optimise environments so midwives, women and families can thrive.

Anna Hennessey, Visiting Research Scholar, Philosophy Department, University of California, Berkeley, and Adjunct Lecturer, Philosophy Department, California State University East Bay. Anna works on the philosophical, religious and artistic dimensions of birth and is writing a book on the way that art and other objects, particularly religious objects, go through a transformative process when used during birth as a rite of passage (Lexington Books, forthcoming). She is also founder of visualizingbirth.org, a website providing women with imagery to use for visualisation during pregnancy, labour and birth. Anna has published and presented widely within the humanities and has her PhD in religious studies, an MA in art history and a BA in philosophy. She is also Co-Chair of the Religions of Asia section for the American Academy of Religion, Western Region, and an editor for the *Chinese America: History and Perspectives* journal.

Joan Gabrielle Lalor, Associate Professor of Midwifery in Trinity College Dublin, Ireland. Joan has worked as a midwife in clinical practice, education and research, and in the last ten years in an academic post. Her PhD developed a theory of adaptation following a diagnosis of a fetal anomaly in pregnancy and her work in this area continues to have impact. Joan is an expert member of the Perinatal Palliative Care Clinical Effectiveness Committee and the Bereavement Guidelines Implementation Group (Ireland) to standardise good practice across maternity care. Joan's other research interests include the concept of the fetal patient, medical health humanities, and legal and ethical issues that emerge in healthcare – in particular, the historical and legal contexts in which court ordered treatment occurs. Joan's research seeks to generate evidence likely to influence governances as women negotiate the structures that surround childbirth and early motherhood.

Céline Lemay, Senior lecturer at Université du Québec à Trois-Rivières in the midwifery program, Canada. Céline started midwifery in the 1980s and was actively involved in the legalisation of midwifery in Québec as an autonomous profession, distinct from medicine and nursing. She has worked in a birthing centre, public institution and midwife-led care for 12 years. Céline is interested in the ethics of practice, clinical reasoning, and ways of knowing and theorising the midwife's paradigm. She is a reviewer of a range of midwifery journals, administrator of l'Ordre des sages-femmes du Québec, and is about to publish a book (in French) on bringing a child into the world: revisiting knowledge and holding together what we count and what counts. Her research methods are rooted in feminism and hermeneutic phenomenology. She is mother of three and grandmother of four.

Luz Stella Losada, along with her husband (Dr José Miguel de Angulo), established MAP International's Bolivian Holistic Community Health and Development programs, which are based on a human rights perspective and child-centered focus. Luz Stella received a master's degree in Health Professions Education (MHPE) from Limburg University, Maastricht, the Netherlands. She has facilitated many programmes focusing on maternal-child health and comprehensive early infancy development with an emphasis on robust brain architecture development. She and her husband co-founded the comprehensive Early Child Development Program for marginal impoverished communities. The programme takes a neuro-psycho-social approach to fostering parental skills. She has co-authored more than a dozen books on human rights protection for child victims of sexual violence and comprehensive early infancy development, including: *12 Strategies for Comprehensive Early Infancy Development*; *Seeds of Change for the New Bolivia of Wellbeing*; *Rediscovering the Amazing and Transcendent Adventure of Pregnancy and Delivery*; and *Parental Competences for Comprehensive Early Infancy Development*.

Ingela Lundgren, Registered midwife and registered nurse, Gothenburg, Sweden. Ingela is a Professor in Reproductive and Perinatal Health at the Institute of Health and Care Sciences, the Sahlgrenska Academy, University of Gothenburg, Sweden. Her position also includes clinical work as a midwife at Sahlgrenska University Hospital, Gothenburg. Ingela completed her education as a midwife in 1986 and has worked with births in standard delivery wards, Birth Centres and homebirths. Her main research interest is about the meaning of childbirth in a woman's life. Ingela is currently involved in several national and international research projects focusing on women's experiences of giving birth and birth from the long-term perspective, support during childbirth by professionals and non-professionals, and the organisation of maternity care. She is an author of books and has written textbook chapters for midwives as well as publishing about research methods.

Jenny Parratt, Fellow of Australian College of Midwives, and Adjunct Associate Professor at Southern Cross University, Australia. Jenny is a mother and has been a registered midwife since 1982. She practised privately for fourteen years, attending homebirths in rural Victoria where she still lives. Now Jenny develops curricula and teaches in online postgraduate programs. Jenny's PhD was entitled 'Feeling Like a Genius: Enhancing Women's Changing Embodied Self During First Childbearing'. Her research methods have a firm philosophical foundation in feminist post-structuralism. Jenny's professional passions are sustaining women's changing embodied self during childbearing and enabling women to have the best possible birth experience. She has written a book, book chapters and journal articles; she is an active journal reviewer and an associate editor of Women and Birth. Currently, Jenny's research focus is on women's experiences and preferences for skin-to-skin contact and breastfeeding during the first 30 minutes after birth.

Gill Thomson, Senior Research Fellow in the Maternal and Infant Nutrition & Nurture research unit, University of Central Lancashire. Gill has been involved in a number of research/evaluation-based projects funded by various Primary Care Trusts, Department of Health and the National Institute of Health Research to explore psychosocial influences and experiences of maternity services, infant feeding issues and support services. She publishes regularly, is an editorial member of high impact journals and is lead editor on two Routledge texts: *Qualitative Research in Midwifery and Childbirth: Phenomenological Approaches* (2011) and *Psychosocial Resilience and Risk in the Perinatal Period: Implications and Guidance for Professionals* (2017). Gill's research interests relate to peer support models of care and psychosocial influences and implications of perinatal care, with a particular focus on factors that impact on maternal mental health. She also has a particular specialism in hermeneutic phenomenology.

FOREWORD

When I was asked to write this foreword, I didn't give it a second thought. I knew immediately that I wanted to be engaged with a book that is so timely, so needed, and edited by two midwives with extensive experience of midwifery, who are known to create a rich tapestry of understanding around the birth of babies.

We are, as I write, going through a revolution in much of the world, and it seems while being pulled in the direction of separation, hostility to people unknown to us, violence and war, lack of respect for environment, and selfish economics, there is a growing counter movement of support and compassion, concern with environment, community growth and development, international understanding, support for human rights, connections between people. Birth can be a great builder of connections.

Similarly, in maternity care, there is a divide. While it must be recognised that improvements in medical treatment and public health measures have saved lives, the over-medicalisation of birth, an approach that focuses on risk and safety, that often seems to treat the woman and her child as having competing interests, where unnecessary interventions are common, and the dignity and autonomy of individual women is often forgotten, is doing great harm.

At the same time, there has been growth of awareness of the need to put women and their babies and families at the centre of care, to wrap them around with services that respond to their needs and that hold them in sensitive respect, and provide alternatives to large-scale standardised hospital maternity care. The development of knowledgeable, skilled, compassionate midwifery has been important to this movement. But this movement forward to more humanised and spiritual care is beset by divides and division, by polarisation and resistance.

Sometimes, when we are faced with jumping a divide so that we retain what is valuable but make changes that are needed, we have to build a bridge that will help us to move on. There are signs of a seismic shift in thinking, not only in the progressive maternity policy seen in many parts of the world, reflecting the fact that birth is more than a medical event, but also in the movement to positive approaches to pregnancy and birth and the early weeks of life expressed by women, men and users of maternity services through writing and social media. Also, the humanisation of birth movement started in Brazil in the late 1990s as a response to brutally medicalised maternity care, is growing, and the basis of human rights around birth is helping to develop care that respects human dignity and autonomy that is respectful to women and their families. There is a growing body of scientific understanding of the complex physiological basis of safe healthy birth that is meshed with the physiological basis of relationship and the growth of mothering and parenting behaviour. We need to bridge the divide to go to the centre.

Childbirth is the physical birth of the relationship between the mother and her baby, the father or other parent and the baby, and a new family. It is a critical time for the formation of secure attachments, the bond of love that will tie the family together and help lay a firm foundation in life. The importance of this relationship runs through these pages together with an exploration of the psychology and physiology, of these transitions. Love, hope and joy, essential aspects of parenting and family relationships, emerge over and over again. Over recent years midwives have worked to create services in which they are enabled to work in relationship with women. This redevelopment of relationship-based midwifery, care mediated through human relationship, is associated with many positive outcomes. Here, in these pages, we can understand the fulfilment midwives may feel when they accompany women and their families on this spiritual journey. In a way midwives model to women what their babies need from them – timely sensitive and compassionate responses to their needs.

Spirituality and Childbirth: Meaning and Care at the Start of Life takes us right to the centre of what pregnancy, birth and the early weeks of life is all about. This is the start of life, a profound event full of possibility and promise, the promise of new life. It is, in what I hope is not too hackneyed a phrase, an everyday miracle. But this book with its focus on practice and meaning takes us beyond these bald statements, and helps us to attune to the spirituality of birth. I have certainly been inspired to think and see anew. It makes connections between all the disparate approaches.

There is a lot that is important in this book. For one thing it is not written in opposition to the biomedical approach, and chapter after chapter makes the point that this is not meant to create false dichotomies. It does, however, lay out very clearly the problems of a progressively technocratic approach that leaves the felt experiential aspects of birth hidden and unspoken, a dangerous impoverished approach. There is a combination of different theoretical approaches and experience, with interesting crossovers. For example, the sociological examination of the current language of birth, the language of fear, of risk, of danger, of measurements that are confined to numbers, helps us to imagine a more positive future in which birth is thought about and spoken about and experienced as a powerful meaningful and spiritual event. This examination will help and inform our practice in a way that upholds the dignity of the woman her baby and her family and highlight how we need to treat everyone with respect.

The meaning of spirituality is teased out; spirituality is wider than religion and is not limited to religious belief. Recently, just before I read this book, in preparing for a major lecture that I am to deliver at a turning point in my life, I suddenly remembered the words of a woman I was midwife to years ago. She lived in social housing in the streets around Wormwood Scrubs prison in London. She had experienced a major complication in her pregnancy and we were talking through how we might approach the doctors so that she could be more involved in decisions about her own care. I had been 'palpating' her abdomen (we need a different term for this!) when she suddenly said, 'You know I keep thinking and thinking about it, I have another person growing inside me and I just can't get over it.' This other person inside the woman is an important theme in the book and must, when you think about it, provoke awe and wonder. It has often struck me that pregnancy and birth and those challenging early weeks of life are undeniably human and practical, messy and challenging while being sacred. It is a combination of earthliness and the divine, this most fundamental transition in life and the world.

So, through *Spirituality and Childbirth: Meaning and Care at the Start of Life*, we are taken into transcendence; we are invited to think about the profound meaning of the experience and the work for those involved. The impact of our approaches, the power of relationship in creating this relationship being born, the power of sensitivity to the needs of the people involved, the power of being in awe of our privilege, can lead directly to a better future. But, our care can also harm badly, creating not only physical and psychic harm but also the harm of reduction and impoverishment of an event that holds such meaning and profound importance.

Spirituality, we are told clearly, is not confined to normal or physiological birth or birth where the outcome is positive. This is not a spirituality of flute music. It is a spirituality that is concerned with relationship, with connections to others and the divine, with personal growth not only from joy but also from loss, adversity and trauma.

I love the way that the principles of effective and high quality care are woven into the spiritual approaches, alongside cutting edge physiological understanding. The different chapter authors bring a variety of perspectives, of deep insight and different streams of academic literature as well as art. I couldn't stop thinking, when I read the chapter based on artistic understanding, about the use of the term 'crowning'. It is of course the term used for crowning a king or queen, but here in this moment, often of searing pain, the women crowns her own child. I had never thought about it like this before. Now I understand the halos!

What can you get from this book? That will depend on you and your perspective on life and the meaning of life. This is important; the approach is not dogmatic, but encourages openness to experience and meaning in the reader, just as in practice we must be open to individual experience and meaning.

For me, I am left with a sense of wholeness, of being brought to the centre, of connections. This is a feeling I have often had as a midwife, often at home or birth centre births but also in busy very technical labour wards too, that my work as a midwife takes me to the centre of the world, the start of everything, this person being born, the partner becoming parent, the family being created, the woman becoming mother. Of course it stands to reason, that we should at every birth and in all our care be aware of the sacred nature of this time, but I don't think we think about it like that very much.

As Susan and Jenny conclude, there are many different ways to practise, but if we are sensitive, compassionate, respectful of human beings, it brings a deeper connectedness that will transcend differences. This approach will help us to understand the journey of birth better, and can take us into the birth of better maternity services and a better world.

I recommend *Spirituality and Childbirth: Meaning and Care at the Start of Life* for anybody concerned with birth. It will help you to think differently and attune you to spiritual meanings. It will challenge and support you to a more holistic approach that recognises the profound significance of this powerful and meaningful event, what is essentially the birth of our future.

Lesley Ann Page CBE

President Royal College of Midwives (UK)
Visiting Professor, Florence Nightingale Faculty of
Nursing and Midwifery, Kings College London (KCL)
Adjunct Professor UTS and Griffith University Australia

Oxford, April 2017

ACKNOWLEDGEMENTS

Any project that is broad, in-depth and as ineffable as spirituality and childbirth touches one's core, one's soul and sense of self. This book is a culmination of heartfelt inspiration and passion – a project that started as a small flame and, when shared with others, became fanned into a vast warm bright light.

We would like to thank all our generous authors who have been so patient in the gestation of this book. With their insight, enthusiasm and energy, and despite many competing personal and professional demands, they have written the most beautiful chapters. We have felt humbled by the way each author brought into words a phenomenon that often resists description by words alone. Yet each author has achieved just that, for which they all need to be congratulated.

We would like to thank the publishers who believed in our vision for this book from the beginning. The world of publishing can be challenging and the help provided has been useful in that journey. We also thank the 'unknown reviewers' who gave the 'permission' to proceed with this project and provided great advice as the book's contents took shape.

I (Susan) would like to thank my husband Toby who has been 'there', always believing, always encouraging. Without his support this project would have been all the more challenging. In the middle of editing this book we moved countries; no easy task! I would also like to thank the community of practitioners and scholars that I have had the good fortune to work and think with over the years across many regions in the world. Their contribution to my thinking and 'feeling' the sense-world of childbirth has been cultivated and nurtured my fascination with spirituality and childbirth. Above all I will always be grateful for each time I have been privileged to be invited to walk alongside a woman and her family at the dawn of new life, however difficult the circumstances may or may not have been at the time – those moments have been wondrous and have altered who I am as a human being.

I (Jenny) would like to thank my husband Mark, who has been on the journey toward this book with me for the past 30 years. His realisation, early in our marriage, that this 'midwifery stuff' is part of who I am led to a great deal of childcare and cooking on his part. But he and the births of our five daughters have been completely involved in my spiritual journey and the birth of this book. They are my inspiration always. I would also like to thank the many colleagues from midwifery and nursing internationally who have contributed to discussions and debate about the meanings of spirituality in relation to birth. You have offered ideas and challenged me in many ways, as well as reinforcing that spirituality is an important topic for maternity caregivers to discuss.

Finally we would like to thank you the reader; you have decided to join us in thinking anew how we are faring in and around childbirth. We are honoured that you want to join us in this incredible unfolding journey of discovery.

PART I

Setting the context

1

INTRODUCTION

Susan Crowther and Jenny Hall

Human civilisation has witnessed changes in the social and cultural context of childbirth. These changes involve continuing modification in symbolism, behaviour, organisation of care and emergence of new value and belief systems. Birth is a unique social and cultural occasion holding meaning for society as a whole and each of us individually. Childbirth practices thus reflect significant cultural conditions and values (Crouch and Manderson 1993). The subsequent influences of these conditions and values on birth experience are dynamic and changeable and reflect social, religious, spiritual and emotional meanings. Birth ideologies, medical or natural, foreground cultural and political discourses revealing the effective dominant beliefs and ideas of a time and place. Over time such values and beliefs form images of the prevailing culture and contribute to the social, emotional and spiritual interpretations of birth. What is unclear is how spirituality in the context of childbirth continues to unfold as part of the human experience of childbirth in the 21st century and whether this needs addressing.

This book focuses on spirituality in and around childbirth. Drawing on a body of published work, unpublished research and our unique perspectives as co-editors along with our chapter authors, this book addresses spirituality at the start of life from a variety of thought-provoking perspectives about how 21st century childbirth is considered. Childbirth in this context refers to an undividable continuum of pregnancy-birth-postnatal; we believe that it is nonsensical to introduce arbitrary divisions between so-called 'trimesters and parts' of the childbirth year.

The topic of spirituality and childbirth has beckoned us both for a long time through personal and professional experiences. As we sought ways of reconciling our inner knowing something meaningful about childbirth and how this can and does influence childbirth practices began to call for us to take action – the result of which was the genesis of this book. But why does spirituality at the start of life need addressing in the 21st century context? Surely we now live in a secular technological society with advances in biomedical research and scientific techniques that have made childbirth, at least in the middle to high income regions, as safe as it has ever been in human history? Of course, that in itself is questionable with the increasing array of iatrogenic consequences emerging due to over-zealous usage of contemporary birth technologies (e.g. Downe 2004, Kitzinger 2012, Gaskin 2011, McAra-Couper, Jones, and Smythe 2010, Stone 2009, Davis-Floyd and Cheyney 2009, Fahy, Foureur, and Hastie 2008, Brodsky 2008, Davis-Floyd 2001). However, in our pursuit of safe childbirth have we lost or perhaps hidden something of experiential significance?

Technological birth, natural or normal birth, and holistic social models as opposed to medicalised models of care are well defined by their protagonists and written about extensively elsewhere. However, dichotomous thinking is unhelpful and only serves to occlude the very phenomenon we are seeking to reveal. We are not setting out to prove one understanding is noble and another approach suboptimal, but suggest that there is an approach now so dominant that it threatens to negate and ignore other understandings about childbirth. We contend that childbirth, especially in the western technological context, has become progressively technocratic leaving the felt experiential aspects hidden and unspoken. Examination of spirituality at the start of life reveals another depth of understanding to childbirth not commonly acknowledged. Our concern is that perhaps we are losing something of existential significance in our technolust[1] orientated human world? Can we really afford to ignore spirituality as human beings in all our activities and experiences? Nicola Slee (2004) suggests that spirituality is unique and deeply personal to each of us and is implicit within humanity. Would this not have implications as we bring our attention to childbirth?

There is emergent evidence that spirituality in and around childbirth is experienced as a personal sense of opening and unfolding of self-awareness and self-knowledge which brings inner strength. Pregnancy and birth appears to draw women into proximity with the divine (sense of 'other') and be transformative (Moloney 2007). Nicola Slee (2004) concurs and found that spirituality in and around childbirth is an opportunity to open to 'divinity' (whatever that may mean for you) in ways that are not possible in other ways. She describes how for many women spirituality is a 'vibrant and manifestly obvious fact' (2004, 2) and found that birth holds potential for women to become realised, liberated and spiritual awakened. Other researchers have found the same suggesting that birth for women can bring deeper awareness of connectedness between self, others and divinity and be a time to become more aware and reflect upon spiritual connection (Jesse, Schoneboom, and Blanchard 2007). Given this emergent evidence revealing the experience of spirituality in and around childbirth the implications for health care professionals working in maternity care are significant.

Health care professionals nationally and internationally are charged with providing holistic and spiritual care. This gestures to the need to explore and highlight the meaningfulness of childbirth and how these meanings inform (or not) contemporary childbirth practices, both for professional and lay persons. Through the following chapters the spiritual significance of childbirth is drawn out so that you are confronted with the apparent paradox of biomedical-technocratic systems and the lived experiences of meaningful encounters that often stir all of us involved with childbirth, both professionally and personally.

Several books have focused on spirituality in health care (e.g. Wright 2005, de Souza, Bone, and Watson 2016) and several book chapters and articles are dedicated to health and spirituality (e.g. Pesut, Fowler, Taylor, Reimer-Kirkham, et al. 2008, Paley 2008, Gilliat-Ray 2003, Tanyi 2002, Cawley 1997). Yet little on childbirth and spirituality. Jenny has previously published 'Midwifery, mind and spirit: emerging issues of care' in 2000, which is now out of print and out of date. Surprisingly we found no other book dedicated to this topic (at least in English up to early 2017). Although there is considerable literature on spirituality at the end of life (i.e. hospice care, palliative care, chaplaincy for the dying) there are no books that draw together global academic researchers and practitioners who have an interest in spirituality at the start of life. We have therefore drawn upon a variety of disciplines to gather a variety of perspectives from midwifery, anthropology, psychology, social sciences, hermeneutics and contemporary religious studies. Each chapter brings a style that is innovative, engaging and invokes reflection on aspects of birth normally taken for granted, ignored or left silenced.

In this collection of edited chapters the art and meaning of childbirth is highlighted and contributes to deeper understandings and appreciation of this significant human experience. Through the chapters we draw attention to the beginning of life; a poignant human journey that holds meaning and significance within and beyond current maternity care systems. The overriding themes that inform this book have evolved over time in dialogue with our chapter authors:

- recognition of spirituality at the start of life (mother, baby, family, community)
- exploration of the notions of holism and spirituality
- spiritual experience and childbirth (health care and non-health care professionals)
- spiritual care in maternity care provision
- childbirth as significant bringing meaning and purpose to life at individual and societal level
- spiritual experience when birth is complex and challenging
- childbirth when there is the juxtaposition of birth and death.

What is evident is that something of significance was happening in and around birth and that to appreciate this required multiple perspectives.

Thinking about spirituality

Given that bounded definitions are not feasible we provide here a starting place for our thinking together about spirituality. As Swinton and Pattison (2010) contend definitions of spirituality are always fluid, various and imprecise. The following is not to be taken as universally agreed interpretations of spirituality but an opportunity to ignite our dialogue with you. We begin by suggesting that spirituality is the quality in our lives that gifts meaning and purpose helping us interpret life's experiences. Spirituality is thus a shared human quality that establishes who we are. In other words, we can no more be alive without physical bodies and minds than without our spirituality. These constituents of our existence are non-hierarchical and mutually inclusive; in other words we would cease to 'be' without spirituality.

If we start with the notion as Ammerman (2013) suggests that spirituality may or may not be connected to religion we are confronted by a possible conundrum. If spirituality can stand alone from religion as now commonly espoused, what is spirituality? The problem with this question is it implies that spirituality is an objective entity, reality or notion. We would say all people are spiritual, physical and psychic beings and aver that spirituality and spiritual experience are part of being human and our everyday human experience manifesting in a multitude of ways in relation to time, place and person. While reviewing the literature for this chapter, key qualities of spirituality and spiritual experience continually addressed us:

- transformative (Paul 2014, Lahood 2007)
- relational presence (Pembroke and Pembroke 2008, Heron 1992, Dyson, Cobb, and Forman 1997)
- wholeness, unity, connection (Wilber 2007)
- relationships, connectedness and relatedness to self, others and divinity (Dyson, Cobb, and Forman 1997)
- integral to our wellbeing (Pesut, Fowler, Taylor, Reimer Kirkham, et al. 2008, Swinton 2001)
- meaning and purpose (Hall 2012, Dyson, Cobb, and Forman 1997)
- creativity, mysticism, imminence *and* transcendence (de Souza, Bone, and Watson 2016)
- religious and secular (de Souza, Bone, and Watson 2016)
- intuition and non-rational (Parratt and Fahy 2008)
- coming home (O'Donohue 2012)
- sacred opening (Moore 1992)
- faith (Smith 1979).

This list of qualities and those who wrote about them is in no way presented as exhaustive; it serves only to draw our focus into the need for an open attitude to the notion. What is striking in the above list is the relational interconnected wholeness that nurtures wellbeing and promotes meaning and purpose in our lives. For some of you reading this book spirituality may be strongly connected to faith. Yet faith and religiosity are not necessarily connected. Faith has been described as

> an orientation of the personality, to oneself, to ones neighbours, to the universe; a total response; a way of seeing whatever one sees, and of handling whatever one handles; a capacity to live a more than a mundane level; to see, to feel, to act in terms of a transcendental dimension.
>
> *(Cantwell and Smith 1979, 12)*

This definition of faith implies a way of being in the world, an orientation that may or may not be connected to religiosity, a way of attuning to the situations we find ourselves in as human beings; such as being in and around childbirth. We would proffer that spirituality therefore is part of all of us whether or not we acknowledge and accept this as part of our human existential experience of who we are. Exploring the literature for a definition of spirituality became a journey of discovery as we came to recognise certain qualities were constantly repeated and highlighted, namely, purpose, self-transcending, meaning, meaningful relationships, love and sense of the holy and sacred.

Thinking about what we mean by 'sacred'

Another term that can cause confusion and challenge us is the notion of sacred. Susan's interpretation is that the sacred lies at the core of our human challenge to connect with nature, life's purpose, sense of and relation to divinity (religious or otherwise) and our unfolding relational meaningfulness in our daily lived-interconnecting experiences. This may be through ritual, prayer, singing, being held in the compassionate free attention of another, being in awe at a sunset, beholding the beauty of art or being at a birth and/or death (as both may come at the same time). To be confronted by the sacred is not solely a religious experience; indeed the sacred may or may not be religious in origin (de Souza, Bone, and Watson (eds) 2016). The sacred experience is often composed of transcendental and imminent earthly embodied encounters. Reason (1993) describes sacred experience as being

> based in reverence, in awe and love for creation, valuing it for its own sake, in its own right as a living presence. It is based in the emotions – zest, joy, passion – that helps life process flow as opposed to the stuck unexpressed emotions that may distort experience.
>
> *(Reason 1993, 278)*

If spirituality involves a quest for the purpose in life and meaning to the project of living, then birth, as a sacred event, can be interpreted as the start of an ongoing journey for the new baby, the parents and family/community. We contend that experiences at the start of life confront us all with something profoundly meaningful yet often inexplicable.

Complexity of writing about spirituality

Researching and attempting to write about ineffability, spirituality and sacred experience is complex and challenging. How birth is 'languaged' (that is the words used to describe and share ideas about birth) in contemporary society are, we would argue, covering something up and denying another dimension of knowing. Words like fearful, risky, dangerous, secular, medical, public and measurable appear dominant in contemporary language about childbirth, inferring that childbirth needs to be clearly defined, bounded and controlled to be safe.

Heidegger (Heidegger 1927/1962) tells us that there is no fixed final 'truth' about any phenomenon but an ongoing un-concealing or uncovering of what is hidden, yet to be known and still to be noticed. This is no less so than when we explore what 'is' childbirth. The beauty of a book like this one, written by multiple authors with many perspectives, is the opportunity to draw our attention to the multiplicity of human spirituality in and around birth whilst remembering that there is always more, always more to know which lies tantalisingly just out of our present gaze of attention. Often we catch a glimpse of something at the edge of our understanding but it just as quickly disappears from our thinking. The task of articulating a phenomenon which resists bounded definitions is challenging in a world that likes to agree labels and definitions. Spirituality defies our need to simplify it into a word or words because spirituality is never the words we label it with; it is always more. So our inquiry into spirituality forever must remain open for further exploration and uncovering.

What we have found is that each chapter author's writing brought new understandings and insight. As editors we provided guidance to content and style of chapters to ensure flow of chapter after chapter. What we received back was a mosaic of human thought and feeling. Each author in this book (including us as editors) came to this topic with differing lenses, perspectives, life experiences and personal and professional beliefs. All these make up who we are and determined what is most important about this topic to us as individuals. This was born out by the unique ways of expressing spirituality through language. We came to realise in our editing of chapters that the phenomenon of spirituality, due to its ineffability and resistance to being pinned down by single phrases, definitions and words, mirrors both universal and individual qualities in an eternal dance. Each author gifted more in their expression of 'spirituality' revealing more and more of the phenomenon.

The editorial process brought new insights and new experiences to the fore in an ever-evolving process as conflicts and readjustments to the new ways of thinking were brought into play. This dialectic 'play' of meaning created a harmony of deepening understandings stemming from the intentions and ideological dispositions of all of us involved in the writing of this book. This meant that we needed to remain both disciplined and focused on the themes of this book as a whole while allowing emerging horizons of understandings to surface from each chapter. Laverty (2003, 10) describes Gadamer's notion of 'horizon' as 'a range of vision that includes everything seen from a particular vantage point ... to have a horizon means being able to see beyond what is close at hand'. Likewise this book has been a process of different horizons fusing revealing new wholeness that was more than the sum of the individual contributions.

From the beginning, editing this book was going to be a journey bursting with myriad points of view; how could it not? From the first publisher's review of the book proposal suggestions for changes and different approaches were debated, agreed and adapted. We had entered a world without hard definable concepts and clearly understood notions, a domain of human experience that was so varied and expansive that it simply could never be fully told in one book.

Attempting to gather snowflakes

To speak of universal qualities and attributes of spirituality is like attempting to catch each snowflake as it falls; even if all snowflakes could be gathered they would soon melt away! Thus the challenge and nonsensicalness of presenting mutually agreed definitions on such an expansive all-encompassing yet unspoken human experience like spirituality is at best futile. Indeed, we maintain that it is wise to simply enjoy the snowflakes as they fall appreciating the majesty of diversity that each delicately crafted snowflake gifted. Likewise each author in this book crafted their own interpretations on the task we set before them. Titles and focuses of chapters evolved over time; authors had dialogues with co-authors and with us as their editors until eventually their unique contributions took shape. We knew that we could have continued polishing and adding more to what we had. Alas deadlines, workloads and wordage allowances enabled us to draw an imaginary line in the sand knowing full well that there will always be more, that each author would always have more to gift, that more chapters could have been added and that more interpretations could have been presented.

Structure and how to read this book

We would invite you to adopt an open attitude of wonder as you read the words of others and allow them to engage with your thinking. Some things will resonate with you; other parts may not. Parts of this book may even resonate on one day but not on another when re-read! Reading with such openness enables the possibility for more to be revealed as you (the reader) bring your thinking, experience (past, present and future possibilities) into a dialogue with each author in this book and the book as a whole.

The book is presented in three parts. Part 1 is concerned with setting the scene and explores the contextual and philosophical nuances of childbirth from several perspectives. Part 2 focuses on the childbirth year; pregnancy, labour and birth, the immediate postnatal period and parenthood. Part 3 attempts to pull the threads of the preceding chapters together in the final chapter. Each chapter has three themes not in any rigid lineal structure but weaved throughout:

1 **Philosophical underpinnings, theoretical frameworks and definitions.** This theme provides an opportunity for you the reader to glimpse into the contextual reality and pre-understandings of the author(s). How authors are positioned in their thinking and experience and how they uniquely address the principles of this book is helpful in understanding each author's interpretations.

2 **Experiences/stories.** These are narratives from research, practice and personal experience. Stories have value in the telling, the hearing and reading. There is a synergy between spirituality and stories that help in our shared meaning making about childbirth. As we hear and read stories we uncover new insights as deeper understandings of ourselves bubble up into consciousness. According to Atkinson (1995) stories provide the language and form to convey meanings about ineffable experiences of life which are often challenging to speak about. Within hearing and reading a story there is the opportunity to transcend out personal concerns and enter, as Atkinson suggests, 'the realm of the sacred' (11). The many stories in this book gift something of value that we feel will contribute to your life narrative about life and birth.

3 **Implications and practical suggestions.** This theme includes plans for going forward, the 'so what?' – for example, what is the potential for further research, future collaborations, practice approaches and health care professional and non-health care education development?

An invitation to thinking together

We wanted this book to provide voice to often unspoken experiences and frequently silenced researchers and practitioners working in and around childbirth, who honour the synergy between spirituality and childbirth. The hope is that this book will provide a source for further research, future collaborations and inform childbirth practice approaches as well as provide reference for health care professional and non-health care education enhancement. Where you arrive after your journey of reading and thinking will be different for each person. That is the marvel of being human – never quite knowing it all. Our invitation is to immerse yourself into an engaged play of thinking and embrace the dialogue with our chapter authors; that is to say, allow yourself to be in thinking conversation with the author's words. In our thinking together meaningful insights can arise contributing to a renaissance of spiritual awareness in and around 21st century childbirth.

Our hope is that the multiple understandings and perspectives shared in the following chapters provoke a deeper appreciation of spirituality and childbirth. The potential for remembering what was forgotten and arrival of new meaningful insights in our shared thinking may offer possibilities hitherto not appreciated. It is hoped that these new insights and remembrances bring possibilities for transforming our experiences, practices and actions in whatever way we find ourselves involved in childbirth.

Note

1 Technolust is the fascination and attraction to constantly new and perceived better technology in all facets of modern life, including advances in around childbirth management and practice approaches – for example, the advent of 3D imaging in pregnancy ultrasound.

References

Ammerman, N.T. 2013. "Spiritual but not religious? Beyond binary choices in the study of religion." *Journal for the Scientific Study of Religion* 52:258–278. doi: 10.1111/jssr.12024.

Atkinson, R. 1995. *The gift of stories: Practical and spiritual applications of autobiography, life stories, and personal mythmaking.* London, CT: Greenwood Publishing Group.

Brodsky, P.L. 2008. *The control of childbirth.* London: McFarland & Company, Inc.

Cantwell, W. and Smith, W.C. 1979. *Faith and Belief.* Princeton, NJ: Princeton University Press.

Cawley, N. 1997. "Towards defining spirituality. An exploration of the concept of spirituality." *International Journal of Palliative Nursing* 3 (1):31–36.

Crouch, M. and Manderson, L. 1993. "Parturition as social metaphor." *The Australian and New Zealand Journal of Sociology* 29 (1):55–72. doi: 10-1177/144078302900104.

Davis-Floyd, R. 2001. "The technocratic, humanistic and holistic paradigms of childbirth." *International Journal of Gynaecology and Obstetrics* 45:S5–S23.

Davis-Floyd, R. and Cheyney, M. 2009. "Birth and the big bad wolf: An evolutionary perspective." In *Childbirth across cultures: Ideas and practices of pregnancy, childbirth and the postpartum*, edited by H. Selin and P.K. Stone, 1–22. New York: Springer.

de Souza, M., Bone, J. and Watson, J. eds. 2016. *Spirituality across disciplines: Research and practice.* Cham, Switzerland: Springer.

Downe, S. ed. 2004. *Normal childbirth: Debate and evidence.* London: Churchill Livingston.

Dyson, J., Cobb, M. and Forman, D. 1997. "The meaning of spirituality: A literature review." *Journal of Advanced Nursing* 26 (6):1183–1188.

Fahy, K., Foureur, M. and Hastie, C. 2008. *Birth territory and midwifery guardianship: Books for midwives.* London: Butterworth Heinemann Elsevier.

Gaskin, I.M. 2011. *Birth matters – a midwife's manifesta.* New York: Seven Stories Press.

Gilliat-Ray, S.. 2003. "Nursing, professionalism, and spirituality." *Journal of Contemporary Religion* 18 (3):335–349. doi: 10.1080/13537900310001601695.

Hall, J. 2012. "The essence of the art of a midwife: Holistic, multidimensional meanings and experiences explored through creative inquiry." PhD, Faculty of Arts, Creative Industries and Education, University of the West of England.

Heidegger, M. 1927/1962. *Being and time.* Translated by J. Macquarrie and E. Robinson. New York: Harper.

Heron, J. 1992. *Feeling and personhood: Psychology in another key*. Thousand Oaks, CA: Sage Publications.

Jesse, E.D., Schoneboom, C. and Blanchard, A. 2007. "The effect of faith or spirituality in pregnancy." *Journal of Holistic Nursing* 25 (3):151–158.

Kitzinger, S. 2012. "Rediscovering the social model of childbirth." *Birth* 39 (4):301–304. doi: 10.1111/birt.12005.

Lahood, G. 2007. "Rumour of angels and heavenly midwives: Anthropology of transpersonal events and childbirth." *Women and Birth* 20 (1):3–10.

Laverty, S.M. 2003. "Hermeneutic phenomenology and phenomenology: A comparison of historical and methodological considerations." *International Journal of Qualitative Methods* 2 (3): Article 3: 1–29.

McAra-Couper, J., Jones, M. and Smythe, E. 2010. "Rising rates of intervention in childbirth." *British Journal of Midwifery* 18 (3):160–169.

Moloney, S. 2007. "Dancing with the wind: A methodological approach to researching women's spirituality around menstruation and birth." *International Journal of Qualitative Methods*, 6(1): Article 7. Available from www.ualberta.ca/~iiqm/ backissues/6_1/ moloney.htm

Moore, T. 1992. *Care of the soul*. New York: Harper Perennial.

O'Donohue, J. 2012. *The four elements: Reflections on nature*. London: Transworld Ireland.

Paley, J. 2008. "Spirituality and nursing: A reductionist approach: Original article." *Nursing Philosophy* 9 (1):3–18.

Parratt, J. and Fahy, K.M. 2008. "Including the nonrational is sensible midwifery." *Women and Birth* 21 (1):37–42.

Paul, L.A. 2014. *Transformative experience*. Oxford: Oxford University Press.

Pembroke, N.F. and Pembroke, J.J. 2008. "The spirituality of presence in midwifery care." *Midwifery* 24 (3):321–327.

Pesut, B., Fowler, M., Taylor, E.J., Reimer Kirkham, S. and Sawatzky, R. 2008. "Conceptualising spirituality and religion for healthcare." *Journal of Clinical Nursing* 17 (21):2803–2810. doi: 10.1111/j.1365-2702.2008.02344.x.

Reason, P. 1993. "Reflections on sacred experience and sacred science." *Journal of Management Inquiry* 2 (3):273–283. doi: 10.1177/105649269323009.

Slee, N. 2004. *Women's faith development: Patterns and processes*. Aldershot: Ashgate.

Smith, W. 1979. *Faith and belief*. Princeton, NJ: Princeton University Press.

Stone, P.K. 2009. "A history of western medicine, labor, and birth." In *Childbirth across cultures: Ideas and practices of pregnancy, childbirth and the postpartum*, edited by H. Selin and P.K. Stone, 41–53. New York: Springer.

Swinton, J 2001. *Spirituality and mental health care: Rediscovering a "forgotten" dimension*. London: Jessica Kingsley Publishers.

Swinton, J. and Pattison, S. 2010. "Moving beyond clarity: towards a thin, vague, and useful understanding of spirituality in nursing care." *Nursing Philosophy* 11 (4): 226–37. doi: 10.1111/j.1466-769X.2010.00450.x.

Tanyi, R.A. 2002. "Towards clarification of the meaning of spirituality." *Journal of Advanced Nursing* 39 (5):500–509. doi: 10.1046/j.1365-2648.2002.02315.x.

Wilber, K. 2007. *Integral spirituality: A startling new role for religion in the modern and postmodern world*. Boston, MA: Shambhala Publications.

Wright, S.G. 2005. *Reflections on spirituality and health*. London: Whurr Publishers.

2

CHILDBIRTH AS A SACRED CELEBRATION

Susan Crowther

Introduction

This chapter explores how childbirth is spiritually experienced and meaningful within society revealing how childbirth has purpose both individually and collectively. The discourse and mood around childbirth internationally is often concerned with risk, morbidity and mortality yet philosophers O'Byrne (2010) and Arendt (1958) infer that childbirth is a celebration of natality and future possibility, not purely avoidance of mortality. This chapter acknowledges birth as both joy and sorrow, birth as the potential for epiphany, peak experience, moments of self-actualisation and a time of remembrance. The notions of Kairos time (sacred felt-time) at birth and meaningful encounters in and around childbirth are introduced with narrative examples. Something lies quiescent in the background of childbirth gesturing to ineffability, the inexplicable, and what is mysterious and awe inspiring.

> It was 3 am when I was awoken to the ring tone of my mobile phone. I heard Sally on the end of the phone breathing heavy telling me it was time. I was her community midwife and we had known each other for several years as she grew her family. I pulled up outside her home gathered my things and walked up the path to her door gazing at the stars in the sky and hearing the sounds of the night; a glorious night to have a baby. Sally was on her knees leaning over the bed with her head buried in pillows. The youngest was awake and playing with his grandfather. Sally's partner, Tom, was pacing and yawning. I leaned over to Sally and said 'I'm here Sally' and arranged my notes and homebirth equipment. I was concerned as I was unable to contact my practice partner because there was no phone signal. The youngest, David, ran in and jumped on me 'Sue, Sue middywife!' then jumped on the bed and began stroking his

mum's arms as she swayed through contractions. Jane, the eldest, was still asleep in the other room. Within a few minutes Sally stood up and declared that she wanted a shower. We all went to the smallest room in the house surrounded by hanging laundry and within minutes Sally was grunting into her throat with a distinctive expulsive eeeeeeer sound. She went onto her knees and pushed involuntarily in the bath as the shower continued to drench us all. Sally then turned over as the water level rose in the bath tub and gave what can only be described as an out of this world pushing sound that switched the mood in the bathroom in an instant. The baby was coming – the head stretching and pushing onto the perineum. I went into midwife overdrive and arranged what I needed close to hand. It was cramped and professionally I was alone. Then a baby boy came into the world underwater. Sally took him into her arms as he took a massive intake of breath. Sally burst into tears saying 'Welcome little one, you're beautiful.' I looked up and saw Tom now with both children sitting on his knees – all three with tears running down their cheeks. David sat on his dad's knee with his mouth open in surprise. I looked up at the door to the bathroom and there stood the grandfather smiling, eyes moist and nodding. Several hours later I drove home feeling a depth of peace with the world as the sun climbed the morning sky.

The above story is taken from my own midwifery practice and is based on real life events. In that bathroom three generations gathered at the dawn of a new life. In a moment, as I leaned over the bathtub to help greet this new life, past met the present and stretched into a future of possibilities. I felt privileged to be part of this and overcome by the intensity of the moment feeling tears run down my cheeks. As I drove home in the early hours of that day I felt the interconnectedness of everything.

This story gestures to a number of qualities that constitute each and every birth which I have had the privilege to have been invited to – whether at home, a birth centre, a hospital and even in the back of cars! Each birth, with and without technology, unfolds in a special felt-space, within an auspicious felt-time, and is always an occasion that is embodied for all and always includes being with others who are near, far, seen and unseen. The above story reveals how birth gathers all these into an event infused with sacred significance and spiritual meaning.

The sacred stirs at the edge of the unspeakable in my midwifery practice and this unspeakable or ineffable quality is mirrored in the literature I have read over the years and found in my own research related to childbirth. Birth is simply brimming with existential qualities and an abundance of meaningfulness that often leaves us spellbound and profoundly touched – if we allow it to. To be in and around birth is an opportunity for transformation. Attempting to come to an understanding about the wholeness of birth in a fragmented way is the antithesis of experiences in and around birth childbirth, whether as a birthing woman or those of us present at birth as healthcare professionals, family and friends.

Ecology of birth

There is a wholeness about childbirth that I to refer to as an 'ecology of childbirth' which unfolds at each birth (Crowther 2016, Crowther 2014). Yet we need to be cautious of naming something. The notion of an 'ecology of childbirth' (see Figure 2.1) and its implications for how childbirth occurs within contemporary maternity systems is used here as a point of departure in our explorations and is not intended to be taken as a fixed and inflexible notion.

According to Haeckel (1876) ecology is the science of relationship of living things/beings and their environments. What is key in this definition of ecology is the significance of relationships. I would contend that ecology in relation to childbirth is concerned with multiple relationships. It is an interrelated phenomenon comprising an embodied[1] quality, a spatial quality that includes felt-space and physical places of birth, a quality of relationality or being with others, a quality of temporality that incorporates Kairos time (explored later in chapter), a dynamic quality of social-political and cultural context e.g. changing policies and practices informing childbirth. Simultaneously every birth includes

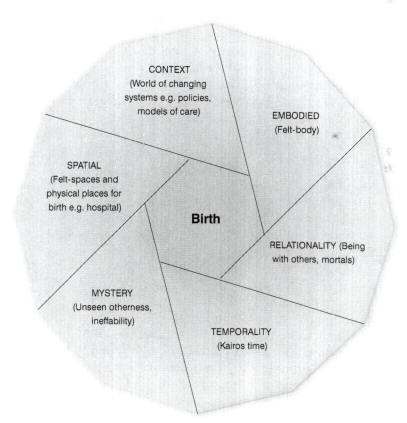

FIGURE 2.1   An ecology of birth

a mysterious unspoken quality unfolding in and around the occasion. This 'ecology of birth' incorporates *all* types of birth in *all* circumstances.

An ecology of birth is a notion built upon the enigmatic description of Heidegger's fourfold[2] (Heidegger 1971/2001a), Smythe et al's (2016) interpretation of the 'good birth' and my own research in relation to the existential qualities of lived-experiences of being at the time of birth (Crowther 2014). Reawakening our collective cognisance of an ecology of birth can bring remembrance of how each birth is potentially a joyful celebration of life and our shared natality. I infer a 'reawakening' as I fear we have forgotten or covered up our original knowing. In this chapter I adopt a phenomenological and philosophical hermeneutic lens informed by the works of Heidegger (1927/1962), Gadamer (2008/1967), Arendt (1958), Dilthey (2002) and O'Byrne (2010) to present a philosophical interpretation of birth as spiritually meaningful.

Being-at-birth

The phenomenological experience of 'being-at-birth' is drawn from my own doctoral work that explored the lived experiences of being at the moment of a baby being born. When I first examined being there at birth four constituent qualities of embodiment, spatiality, relationality and temporality were revealed. These initial interpretations were not the sole qualities of our human experience at birth. These initial interpretations have now evolved into deeper understanding and expanded into an ecology of birth as depicted in Figure 2.1 and will be revisited throughout this chapter.

Embodied experiences

The rationale for using hyphens in 'being-at-birth' is to foreground the unifying quality of the phenomenon, thus 'being-at-birth' signals not how we are 'in' the event of birth, but how we 'are' the unfolding events at birth. This is no less true than when referring to embodied experiences. My study uncovered myriad embodied experiences at the time of birth such as the smiling and tears of the family in the story above. Brenda, an obstetrician, shares how it is to touch a baby for the first time at a caesarean section:

> As soon as I reach in and can touch the baby, I feel excited as I get to be the very first one to touch it! I reach in and it's this first connection with the baby. As soon as my hand goes in and touches the baby I feel a kind of transition. It's hard because I'm constantly balancing between the medical bit and the connection.
>
> *(Crowther 2014, 160)*

Touch invokes a powerful moment of transition for Brenda amidst the technological context of a surgical event. When Brenda touches the baby for the first time a special connection is made, an intimate relationship comes into being between her and the unborn baby. The moment is charged with profound intimacy despite the context. According to Merleau-Ponty (1962/2002) to touch is to be touched; it is a shared communication through the body. This touch moves reciprocally. The baby for the first time feels physically touched by someone outside of the womb. The baby and surgeon are instantly thrown into a mutual tactile encounter. Both human beings in the moment sense themselves in this embodied exchange – an encounter both physical and ontological. In that moment of tactile intimacy two worlds connect and experience one another in a moment of imminence and transcendence.

My research revealed how birth comprises a totality of bodily senses; touching, holding, smelling, seeing, and hearing. Visceral emotional affects such as weeping, smiling and shaking appeared in the gathered birth stories that pointed to something profound and unexplainable. It is as if these powerful sensual and ontological embodied responses burrow deep within our corporal structure, as Heidegger suggests 'down to the last muscle fibre and hidden molecule of hormones' (1971/2001a, 232) and beyond into transcendental experience. Merleau-Ponty's (1962/2002) thesis contends that the body is the primary medium of all perception. We are thus constantly embodied within the world and this is no less so than at birth. Experiences at birth show how birth physically and feelingly reaches out to us and gifts something of significance beyond and within the constraints of our individual experiences. Likewise, the spatial experience of birth is unique and meaningful.

Spatial experiences

Birth place is often referred to in terms of physical structures such as home, hospital or birth centre. Conversely the notion of birth space or atmosphere is the feeling dimension of place, an attuned space, a lived-space which is not necessarily connected to physical places (Crowther 2013). This is not to deny the significance of places of birth. Yet ongoing debates and research agendas concerning place of birth are often ideologically polarising and reveal little about spiritual meaningfulness and sacred significance of different birth spaces. Leaving the debates about birth place to others I focus on the lived experiences of such places of birth and draw our attention to 'felt-space at birth'.

Heidegger refers to this aspect of spatiality as 'directionality' – a space perceived differently according to situation and our ways of attuning to it. The surrounding physical world at birth blends and integrates with the felt-space contributing to an ecology of birth. A place of birth is thus not defined solely as hospital or home, but rather feeling safe, friendly, warm, fearful, impersonal, intimate, joyful and sacred. Birth space can thus be a felt space that is spiritually meaningful, holding sacred significance. Simone, a midwife, describes how this felt-space at birth transcends the clinical hospital physical environment:

> Every time I go into a hospital and it's very clinical and sterile and clean, there's still a part of me that says, 'Even though this is a hospital, this is a sacred place because life is brought into the world here, new life emerges here, therefore there has to be something special about that place, something sacred.'
>
> *(Crowther 2014, 167)*

The distinction in experiential terms is that physical place and felt space coexist yet are equally important parts of the whole experience. Embodied and spatial experiences are not divided or separate but are in an interconnected relational whole; they are within the interiority of each other.

Relational experiences

Studies have revealed that the environment of birth is at once integral to the relational engagement and connection of others at birth (e.g. Bergum and Van Der Zalm 2007). This gestures to the relationality at birth and how birth gathers others far, near, seen and unseen into intimate nearness. To be in the world is always to be with-other, for, as Heidegger reminds us, we are never alone: 'The world is always the one that I share with Others' (1927/1962, 155). Birth and being born is thus always in some way to be gathered with-others near and far.

Gathering appears to unfold over the process of each birth intensifying around the moment when a baby is born. Others, maternity care providers, friends, family, even community members, come to birth in anticipation of something special, knowing that birth is significant whatever the outcome. Feeling privileged to be at birth was a theme repeatedly mentioned in my own study. Participants reported feeling honoured, privileged and enjoyed being there when a new infant(s) was arriving.

The advent of a new human being appears to act as a clarion call to others to be near, to help, to gather and greet a new baby. Birth acts as a mobilisation of others into action, everyone answering that call come with an array of responsibilities, skills, needs and differing perspectives (Crowther, Smythe and Spence 2014). Despite these outward differences among parents, midwives and obstetricians, they come together at the occasion of each birth in a special gathering. John, a father, highlights this gathering quality:

> My Mum came up and she stopped in. Then my wife's sister came. It was a bit of a family event starting to brew. Then my wife's other sister came with one of her friends! They all come round because they were excited that baby would soon be here.
>
> *(Crowther 2014, 179)*

John reveals how a growing mood of intimate inclusiveness occurs as birth approaches. Others leave their everyday lives to be near because something special, momentous is about to happen. This is paradoxically an intimate yet public expression of being alive that inspires a need for closeness. Tui, a grandmother, describes this communal occasion as jubilant about the new baby:

> There was this lovely kind of parade down the street. People were waving out their windows and cheering! It was lovely. I remember feeling just warm and exciting. It was great with everyone there, lots of little kids.
>
> *(Crowther 2014, 182)*

Like a warm fire in winter bringing others together around the family hearth for warmth and light so too John and Tui describe how birth gathers.

Berg, Ólafsdóttir and Lundgren (2012) showed the importance and significance of relationships creates an affirming space at birth. However, are pre-formed relationships a determining factor in spiritual meaningfulness and sacred significance at birth? Are prior relationships essential to attune to this specialness at birth? Not necessarily. Being at birth was shown to be special in and of itself. Even when birth is among others with no prior relationship the choice to attune to a special mood at birth remains (Crowther, Smythe and Spence 2014). Something about birth seems to gather others near into a shared space and embodied experience. Even being physically present at the moment of birth is not essential to be part of this gathering. My study revealed how others gather from afar in their feelings and aspirations. For example, a mother explains how a she made a phone call to her father who lived far away. As she spoke of this important phone call she wept. The power of the occasion reaches out and touches beyond the immediacy of the birth space – a moment in time that seemingly overflows with temporal significance.

Temporal experiences: Kairos time

My study revealed how something in the moment at birth changes. As Merewether (2013) aptly describes, 'there is a light that comes into the room when a baby is born'. This moment, or moments, in time when a baby is born gestures spiritual meaning and sacred significance:

Simone [midwife] says it is a moment of 'beautiful naturalness, a universal happiness in the room'.

Carol [obstetrician] always feels 'happiness in the room when the baby arrives'.

Lorna [mother] remembers this moment as gifting a 'precious jewel, beyond special, a moment of grace'.

Diane [midwife] describes the moment as beyond words 'an oooh feeling, a whoa or whoo moment!'.

Karl [father] speaks of a mesmerising quality: 'It is just "woo", just watching and listening, just looking at him, focused right in, magnetised.'

Seemingly birth unfolds in a moment of time which can harbour inexplicable and unspoken mystery that captivates and intoxicates. Time is a complex experiential quality of each and every experience. Clock time as a lineal process of structuring and controlling birth was explored by (Downe and Dykes 2009). Clock time is lineal in nature such as the ticking of seconds one to the next, never repeated, always in a forward direction. Cyclic time is akin to the seasons of the year and menstrual cycles. Maialogical time is the intimate time as mother and baby come together in relationship (Dykes 2007). Yet these interpretations of time do not describe fully the quality of time at birth. Time at birth gestures to another quality of time that I have reported more fully elsewhere – a Kairological or Kairos time (Crowther, Smythe and Spence 2015). The qualities of Kairos time include:

- ever new possibilities
- a critical, opportune moment
- a time like no other
- being transformative
- peak experience
- being visible and invisible
- being in fullness of our Being
- coming home
- interconnectedness
- overflowing meaningfulness.

If you now think back to the birth story at the start of this chapter and subsequent quotes in this chapter you may see how Kairos consistently reveals itself as a special quality of time in around childbirth. Perhaps you can feel and appreciate the depth and vastness of meaning overflowing when a new human baby joins us? Even if you have never been physically present at birth; ponder now what that may be like. For myself and many others being at birth is a unique moment in human life: an experience unparalleled in its generosity to gift such penetrating intimacy. As a colleague who had had 40 years of midwifery experience said to me, 'When I drive home after a birth I feel I love the world!' Perhaps this intimate touch gifts a trace of something beyond our everyday mundane lives?

Kairos time at birth draws near the ineffability of life felt in a mood of wonder, openness and deep interconnectedness. To be thrown into this felt-time is to be touched by potent imminent and transcendent qualities – 'imminent' meaning our individual visceral responses and how birth directly inspires us personally. Transcendental meaning infers more than our individualised experiences gesturing to otherness and our shared knowingness that is both within and beyond ourselves. Such meaning thus epitomises our connectedness and interrelatedness across time, places and people (whether seen, unseen, near and far).

These temporal connections may be more emphasised in different cultural cosmological belief systems based on ancestral worship and reverence. For such cultures it would be less problematic to articulate ancestral reverence than for many Anglo-Saxon cultures. For example, most New Zealand Māori have a deep reverence for their ancestors because 'Whakapapa', or genealogy, is a fundamental principle that permeates their whole culture.[3]

By revealing the above four qualities (embodied, spatial, relational and temporal) within experiences of being at birth we begin to foreground a quality of mystery at birth that is transformative.

Birth as transformative experience

Transformative experiences in and around childbirth hint at something shared and collective. At times this transformative experience is unconsciously known and tacit, yet at once spiritually meaningful. Joy at birth as a potent mood turns us towards and awakens us to something significant at birth. The nature of this awakened transformative experience may come 'all at once' and 'gradually change us'. For example, peak experiences appear to catapult us into different awareness with new understandings recognisable to self and others. Maslow (1964) coined the term 'peak experience' to describe moments of joy in everyday experience. Birth has been described as the happiest moments in life, highlighting peak experiences which manifest in a shared joy wherein individual experiences unify with others as described earlier in this chapter. Simultaneously experiences of birth have been described as a powerful self-actualising experience for mothers (Cheyney 2011, Lokugamage 2011) and fathers (Lahood 2007). Peak experiences do not have a lineal progression as with the movement to self-actualisation yet both emerge from experiential data about being at birth. What is evident is that an experience of self-actualisation and peak experiences are connected to meanings central to birth itself. In other words birth can provide meaning, fulfilment of purpose and be personally transformative for all whether as a peak moment in time of overwhelming joyful experience or a gradual process of being self-actualised. Paul (2014) defines a personally transformative experience as:

> life-changing in that it changes what it is like for you to be you. That is, it can change your point of view, and by extension, your personal preferences, and perhaps, even change the kind of person that you are at least take yourself to be ... substantially revising your core preferences or revising how you experience being yourself ...
>
> *(Paul 2014, 16)*

The personally transformative experience of being at births certainly resonates with my own experience as a midwife and what I have repeatedly witnessed working with parents and colleagues. Deciding to become a midwife in the early 1990s seems a world apart from the lived reality of midwifery I experience today. The choice at the time could never have been made on the rational choice of knowing the full extent of what it would be like to be a midwife.

Being a midwife has radically changed how I experience who I am both epistemologically (knowing how I come to know anything) and personally in ways that are impossible to rationally understand. Making the choice to be a midwife and predict how my life would unfold after that choice was not possible. I have been transformed by my multiple experiences of being at births which have fundamentally altered my professional and personal outlook on life in ways I would never have imagined prior to the choice to enter a degree course in midwifery. Likewise, for a birthing woman the transformative experience of becoming a parent may leave pre-birth desires and assumptions about life forever transformed in unknown ways. As Paul (2014) continues:

> [Y]ou face a certain kind of ignorance: ignorance about what it will be like to undergo the experience and ignorance about how the experience will change you.
>
> *(Paul 2014, 32)*

I remember the looks of revelation on a friend's face when assisting me at a mutual friend's homebirth. Within months the friend who assisted me applied to be a midwife and never looked back on her career change. We never know how each birth will affect us, touch us and change us. Being at birth can be profoundly transformative, opening us to peak and self-actualising experiences that are significantly spiritual in nature leading into areas of life not previously considered, desired and known to us. Often these experiences gesture towards a shared quality that transcends the concerns of our individual lives.

Shared natality

At each birth, we are confronted with the majesty of a continuum of life begetting life that reminds us of our interconnectedness with others – past, present and future; as a Māori grandmother explained to me, 'To be at birth is to welcome the past which meets the future in the present moment.' Kairos time, as described earlier, is a conjoining of past, present and future. It is a time in our lives of profound connections. To be attuned to our shared natality is to be 'grounded in the present moment, supported by the past that is arriving and the openness of a future that is calling' (Todnes and Galvin 2010, 4). Birth thus reaches out and touches us in Kairos gifting something unseen and invisible; a numinous encounter with life's shared mysterious continuance.

The philosophical notions of generation (Dilthey 2002) and natality (Arendt 1958, O'Byrne 2010) are, I would contend, central to the meaning of birth for each of us. There is a flow of life generation to generation which gestures towards continuous possibility, hope and creativity as reflected in Arendt's thesis of natality and Dilthey's intergenerational journey of existence. Their theses hint at how each birth is meaningful. Dilthey's concept of generation is embodied, social, historical and political pointing to a unifying wholeness. This intergenerational experience of connectedness for birthing mothers has been highlighted elsewhere (Carter 2009).

Our shared natality is our collective experience at each birth when we accept the invitation and open ourselves to meet and embrace the great mystery of being alive. A baby brings possibility for newness, a life to be lived, an unfolding potential for actualising dreams yet to be dreamt and realised. Arendt (1958) reminds us birth is a miracle that holds the potential to positively progress the world. Birth is an event in human life that lays bare our nature, a nature which constantly unfolds new beginnings and reveals to us our ability to be beginners of something new. Our shared natality is an innate human condition that reminds us that we are both natal beings and mortal beings. As one midwife after 35 years in practice said to me: 'To understand birth this way is to come to know birth as sacrament.' It is about awakening to our shared relationship to an extraordinary moment of magic and transformation:

> Birth is the primary numinous event. It is our major metaphor for life and coming into being. We talk about birth of the universe ... it is how the world came into being. It is the first act of magic – physical testament to the continuity of human and all life.
>
> *(Razak 1990, 168)*

Every story needs a beginning; each life needs to be born. Each birth is testament of our shared innate mystery of being alive, a mystery that hints at the infinite unknown that stretches out before birth. Kairos at birth is thus a moment bringing us face to face with an enigmatic mystery at the centre of our being; from where and to where is our origin? Science may help us understand where and how we arrive physically yet 'that we are here remains mysterious ... invites question and frustrates our attempts to provide answers' (O'Byrne 2010, 20). As O'Donohue (2012) poetically reminds us a 'baby is a creature fresh from eternity' (29) and beyond our limits of understanding.

We are not the centre of birth, we are part and whole of the experience. The moment of birth is unable to be broken into parts; it is always an ecological process involving interweaving relationships with others, environments and what we bring. Birth is thus an interconnected wholeness, our shared history and our commonality; it is a dynamic emergent ecology and testament to life's unending creativity. To witness birth is to be fascinated and inspired and filled with embodied gratitude in our tears, smiles, gentle voices and tender touching, as Tui (grandmother) states it is 'like having a smile all over your body that spreads and doesn't go away' (Crowther 2014, 234). It is a moment of sacred celebration.

Childbirth as sacred celebration

Seemingly childbirth beckons and gathers others near, gifting the possibility to 'see', 'meet' and 'connect' with each other anew. Birth is thus symbolic and self-evident of beginnings that are transformative. It is not just a baby being born but others are being reborn into new relationships. Birth invokes a gathering, makes community; draws us nearer and authenticates a truly being-with unlike most other experiences in life. In our togetherness at that precious yet vulnerable moment we are spellbound by life's continuing magnificence. If we open ourselves at birth to the celebratory quality of the occasion, we experience a joyful unifying phenomenon inducing spiritual feelings. Spiritual meaning and sacred significance at birth is shared beyond the birthing room. Each birth is a remembrance of our continuance into hitherto unknown possibilities:

> When imagination is allowed to move to deep places, the sacred is revealed. The more different kinds of thoughts we experience around a thing and the deeper our reflections go as we are arrested by its artfulness, the more fully its sacredness can emerge.
>
> *(Moore 1992, 289)*

I would urge us all to ponder deeply and attune to the sacredness at birth in all circumstances. The dynamic social-political and cultural context of birth informs much of what we do. Have you noticed how protocols and policies fade as the birth experience fully engages us? This is not to deny the purpose of practice guidance. At birth things can and do go wrong. There are times when birth is experienced as dread and misery, and times when biomedical interventions save and improve lives. At such times birth's mystery remains yet is often covered over and hidden (Crowther, Smythe and Spence 2014). This does not diminish the wonder of birth. What I point to here is how each birth can be meaningfully experienced in all situations – e.g. the homebirth and the elective caesarean section. Is one of these births any less significant and meaningful? As Liz Smythe and colleagues suggest, a 'good birth' is more than the type of birth (Smythe et al. 2016). What is highlighted in this chapter is how birth is an existential transformative and uplifting experience that has for the most part been hidden and forgotten in the current context. Childbirth as sacred celebration needs to be foregrounded and guide our actions in all circumstances.

Towards an ecology of birth

It is evident that false dichotomies and silo thinking are unhelpful in understanding the ecological wholeness of birth. Dichotomous and polemic attitudes that inform much of the context of birth are the antithesis of spirituality and risk covering up something of significance and meaning. My fear is that what is now known becomes forgotten, and far more concerning for us all, we collectively forget that we have forgotten! If such a time comes, spiritual and sacred experience at birth will become solely personal and left unspoken, perhaps relegated to what is least important in contemporary childbirth. This is apparent in many of the behaviours and discourses amongst maternity care providers where services are devoid of relational models of care and human experiences are not prioritised. Despite often feeling inhibited due to contextual demands of the systems in which we practice something extraordinary at birth continually calls us to 'let our guard down'. This can be especially challenging when births are complex.

Sacred celebration may be delayed due to necessary interventions and circumstances yet joy can still awaken and be anticipated. This requires tact and attuning to events beyond the practical urgent actions undertaken (Crowther, Smythe and Spence 2014). This is a message of hope for those who find themselves completely positioned in technology or trauma who may feel they are bereft of meaningful experiences at birth. While I would not deny the usefulness and necessity of technology at birth, caution is required lest technology covers up something of significance at birth: 'Whatever trust has been built up, perhaps over generations, is fragile to the winds of change' (Smythe et al. 2016, 30). This vulnerability needs to be acknowledged so that we safeguard childbirth from narrow reductionist perspectives that diminish our intergenerational trust in childbirth thus hampering an ecology of birth. It is crucial that we honour the ecological wholeness of each birth as a time of shared celebration.

Context holds power and can undermine our best intentions. Selin and Stone (2009) contend that birth culture, particular in the west, has become so entangled with risk avoidance strategies that it is in peril of being reduced to a 'sterile, safe, vacant experience' (xv). McIntosh (2012) also reminds us that how a society interprets birth is fundamental to how a society functions. Allowing birth to be construed as anything but celebratory, meaningful and significant would be a travesty. Authoritative obstetric and indeterminate knowledge are both part of contemporary birth yet meet in an uneasy co-existence. Technology should not be telling us what birth 'is' but assisting us to hold birth safely when required enabling spiritual meaning and sacred significance to surface. We need to collectively reclaim something special at birth by sheltering the celebratory experience.

Birth should not be hurried and rushed for fiscal, philosophical/clinical orientation, buried under workloads or managerial reasons. The current reality of many maternity systems juxtaposed to often unspoken spiritual transformative experiences at birth are incongruent. Collectedly we need to pay closer attention to the specialness of birth and appreciate the 'celebratory over the clinical' (Cheyney 2011, 535). Do those at birth have a responsibility to nurture and enable sacred celebration to flourish? I appreciate that birth can become mundane when health care providers are there at one birth after another yet I would urge a revolution of services in which we can all work in congruence with the sacred transformative experiences. What if we do not address this? Does a loss of meaning and purpose in and around birth leave mothers bereft of something important on their journey to motherhood? There is a pressing need to attend to the wholeness of birth. We all need to re-evaluate society's shared meaning of natality and move towards systems of care that support an ecology of birth.

Practice implications

Sensitivity at birth awakens and frees spiritual meaning and brings it into presence. Yet at times idle chatter, clearing equipment, changing of shifts, entry of unknown others, knocking on the door or using a mobile phone can and does disrupt birth. For example, midwives dashing and rushing in and out can create an atmosphere that lacks calm (Huber and Sandall 2009). It is not only what we do at birth that is important; it is also how we are being there. Peak experiences at birth are supported when there is midwifery spiritual presence, empathy and kindness (Moloney and Gair 2015). Moloney and Gair contend that without such sensitivity and relational depth mothers can be left feeling traumatised and spiritually distressed after birth. Their conclusions highlight once more the significance of relationships and being with others in sensitive ways. Other chapters in this book draw the significance of this out further.

Many families, midwives and obstetricians already know that birth is profoundly significant and meaningful yet they can act insensitively at this precious time. We need to question whether our current maternity systems, practices and ways of being safeguard birth as sacred celebration or not. There are many practitioners working tirelessly to safeguard the sacred at birth and I would like to exonerate those who have the courage to continually notice and celebrate the sacred at birth wherever they practice. Although their example is a beacon of hope in the discordant discourses challenging modern maternity systems, they need to be heard and appreciated otherwise their light will diminish. For any ecological system to survive relationships between living beings and their environment needs to be nourished and enabled to flourish.

Conclusion

Birth as sacred celebration is revealed in this chapter through an ecology of birth. I have revealed how birth is brimming with spiritual meaning and sacred significance and call for us to foster gentleness, tenderness and humility at birth. Those at birth need to preserve and protect the ineffable qualities at birth with respect and reverence. Even in busy maternity care we can be humbled by mystery. Opening ourselves to the possibility of a sacred mood at birth brings us recognition of something of significance that calls out to us silently in the habitual turbulence of modern maternity care. This is something treasured that we must safeguard so that it continues to 'be'.

If we treat the moment of birth with carelessness and brutishness we risk losing the rarity of the gift of a Kairos moment, a gift that calls us to a threshold in which we can dwell in delight and where the invisible comes into presence. It is a moment that celebrates our shared remembrance of natality as life begetting life. Each birth brings hope and possibilities of better tomorrows. Birth nears the world of our shared natality by shining a light on the occasion and assails us deeply touching us in a timeless moment conveying our unified existence beyond institutional structures, discourses, and social and professional differences. When we are confronted by the intense directness of our shared human lived experiences at birth a mood and memory of something close awakens. In that moment, there is an apparent choice to turn towards the mystery or not. If we turn and attune to the mystery we at are at once startled by what was known but unspoken.

Attuning to this remembrance beckons us to be tactful and safeguard an ever-unfolding ecology of childbirth; an ecology interwoven with spirituality through and through. Everything coalesces at birth revealing an ecological living system that needs nurturing to survive. Foregrounding spirituality in this way hopefully provokes our collective re-imagining of birth in the 21st century. To begin, just listen and allow yourself to feel. Natality's sacred celebratory call continuously whispers in the corridors and rooms of our hospitals, birth centres, communities, homes, midwifery and medical schools.

Epilogue

This chapter opened with a birth story and ends with a poem in honour of the many births I have attended as a midwife.

> Suddenly …
> now I see the connection
> with life's eternal beating heart
> I stand in awe
> Tactile warmth and silky hands
> scent of life's bodily fluids
> the beauty of life's first breath and cry!
> Relief passes over me
> Apgar scores and warm towels –
> must note the time!
> The clock hangs on the wall in a timeless moment
> In and beyond time I gather
> with-others I belong
> smiling with tears of joy flowing
> I expand out into space within and without earth's containing places
> I touch and become touched by messenger of joy
> She comes to remind me
> that sweet possibility of
> new beginnings, of
> ancestors providing new tomorrows
> In a sudden treasured moment
> I'm found home; reminded of who I am
> As inheritor I retain a trace
> I come to know – remember
> how we together belong in life's holy constancy

(Crowther 2014, 250)

Notes

1 'Embodied experiences' refers to how the body is the medium of our perceptions (Merleau-Ponty 1962/2002). Experience and bodily sensorial sensations are thus inseparable. For example a joyful experience is both our material body, such as tears of joy, as well as the lived experiencing of the joy. As Heidegger (2001b) contends we body our experiences, that is to say we embody them.
2 Heidegger's (1971/2001a) philosophical notion of the fourfold is a central aspect of how we dwell as human beings in all situations we find ourselves. The fourfold has four components: earth and sky, divinities and mortals, which are an inseparable unity that cannot be divided into separated components. Each component is interconnected and in the interiority of the other. Heidegger claims that human beings are not only a being in the world, but are always part of this fourfold. For further description read Heidegger's (1971/2001a) *Poetry, language, thought* (full reference given at end of chapter).
3 Any reading on Māori culture is my own interpretation. From my understanding there are two broad main differences in worldview: a western individualism that was juxtaposed to the Māori collective living that is more interconnected and less hegemonic with a spirit-world consciousness that informs Māori Tikanga (values/ customs and rules). The intention here is not to delve into Māori beliefs as I am not Māori, have not been immersed in Māoritanga (Māori culture) and remain largely naive about Māori culture and history. Reference to ancestral cultures in this section is simply to provide a wider context.

References

Arendt, H. 1958. *The human condition*. Chigago, IL: University of Chicago Press.

Berg, M., Ólafsdóttir, O.A. and Lundgren, I. 2012. "A midwifery model of woman-centred childbirth care – in Swedish and Icelandic settings." *Sexual and Reproductive Healthcare* 3 (2):79–87. doi: 10.1016/j.srhc.2012.03.001.

Bergum, V. and Van Der Zalm, J. eds. 2007. *Motherlife: Studies of mothering experience*. Alberta, Canada: Pedagon Publishing.

Carter, S.K. 2009. "Gender and childbearing experiences: Revisiting O'Brien's dialectics of reproduction." *NWSA Journal* 21 (2):121–143.

Cheyney, M. 2011. "Reinscribing the birthing body: Homebirth as ritual performance." *Medical Anthropology Quarterly* 25 (4):519–542. doi: 10.1111/j.1548-1387.2011.01183.x.

Crowther, S. 2013. "Sacred space at the moment of birth." *The Practising Midwife* (December):21–23.

Crowther, S. 2014. "Sacred joy at birth: A hermeneutic phenomenology study." Unpublished PhD, Faculty of Health and Environemental Sciences, Auckland University of Technology.

Crowther, S. 2016. "Towards an ecology of birth." Royal College of Midwives Annual Conference, Harrogate International Centre, UK, 19–20 October 2016.

Crowther, S., Smythe, L. and Spence. D. 2014. "Mood and birth experience." *Women and Birth: Journal of the Australian College of Midwives* 27 (1):21–25. doi: 10.1016/j. wombi.2013.02.004.

Crowther, S., Smythe, L. and Spence. D. 2015. "Kairos time at the moment of birth." *Midwifery* 31:451–457. doi: http://dx.doi.org/10.1016/j.midw.2014.11.005.

Dilthey, W. 2002. *Formation of the historical world in the human sciences*. Translated by Rudolf A. Makkreel and Frithjof Rodi. Edited by Rudolf A. Makkreel and Frithjof Rodi, *Selected works/Wilhelm Dilthey*; v.3. Princeton, NJ: Princeton University Press.

Downe, S. and Dykes. F. 2009. "Counting time in pregnancy and labour." In *Childbirth, Midwifery and Concepts of Time*. Edited by C. McCourt, 61–83. London: Berghaun Books.

Dykes, F. 2007. *Breastfeeding in hospital: Mothers, midwives, and the production line*. New York: Routledge.

Gadamer, H.G. 2008/1967. *Philosophical hermeneutics*. Translated by David E. Linge. Edited by David E. Linge. London: University of California Press.

Haeckel, E.H.P.A. 1876. *The history of creation: Or the development of the earth and its inhabitants by the action of natural causes*. Translated by E.R. Lankester. Vol. 2. London: H.S. King and Son.

Heidegger, M. 1927/1962. *Being and time*. Translated by J. Macquarrie and E. Robinson. New York: Harper.

Heidegger, M. 1971/2001a. *Poetry, language, thought*. Translated by A. Hofstadter. New York: HarperCollins.

Heidegger, M. 2001b. *Zollikon seminars: Protocols – Conversations – Letters*. Translated by F. Mayr. Edited by Medard Boss. Evanston, IL: Northwestern University Press.

Huber, U.S. and Sandall. J. 2009. "A qualitative exploration of the creation of calm in a continuity of carer model of maternity care in London." *Midwifery* 25 (6):613–621. doi: 10.1016/j.midw.2007.10.011.

Lahood, G. 2007. "Rumour of angels and heavenly midwives: Anthropology of transpersonal events and childbirth." *Women and Birth* 20 (1):3–10.

Lokugamage, A. 2011. *The heart in the womb*. London: Docamali Limited.

Maslow, A. 1964. *Religions, values and peak experiences*. Columbus, OH: State University Press.

McIntosh, T. 2012. *A social history of maternity and childbirth: Key themes in maternity care*. London: Routledge.

Merewether, J. 2013. *Heart and hands: A history of the struggle to protect healthy childbirth in Australia*. Australia: Go Girl Productions.

Merleau-Ponty, M. 1962/2002. *The phenomenology of perception*. London: Routledge Classics.

Moloney, S. and Gair, S. 2015. "Empathy and spiritual care in midwifery practice: Contributing to women's enhanced birth experiences." *Women Birth* 28 (4):323–328. doi: 10.1016/j.wombi.2015.04.009.

Moore, T. 1992. *Care of the soul*. New York: Harper Perennial.

O'Byrne, A. 2010. *Natality and finitude*. Bloomington, IN: Indiana University Press.

O'Donohue, J. 2012. *The four elements: Reflections on nature*. London: Transworld Ireland.

Paul, L.A. 2014. *Transformative experience*. Oxford: Oxford University Press.

Razak, A. 1990. "Toward a womanist analysis of birth." In *Reweaving the world: The emergence of ecofeminism*. Edited by I. Diamond and G.F. Orenstein, 165–172. San Francisco, CA: Sierra Club Books.

Selin, H. and Stone, P.K. eds. 2009. *Childbirth across cultures: Ideas and practices of pregnancy, childbirth and the postpartum, Science across cultures: The history of non-western medicine*. New York: Springer.

Smythe, E., Hunter, M., Gunn, J., Crowther, S., McAra Couper, J., Wilson, S. and Payne, D. 2016. "Midwifing the notion of a good birth: a philosophical analysis." *Midwifery* 37:25–31. doi: 10.1016/j.midw.2016.03.012.

Todres, L. and Galvin, K. 2010. "'Dwelling-mobility': An existential theory of well-being." *International Journal of Studies Health and Well-being* 5(3):1–6. doi: 10.3402/qhw.v5i3.5444.

3

RITUAL AND ART IN A PHILOSOPHY OF BIRTH

Anna Hennessey

Introduction

My academic work on birth is inspired by the way that images and visualization coalesced for me in the experience of birthing my first child, Kieran, in 2009. In that instance, the particular image that became crucial to the birth was a Chinese Daoist print called the *Neijing tu*, or the Diagram of Internal Pathways (Figure 3.1). The image depicts an imagination of an internal landscape, including mountains, rivers, and fields, that encompasses the human body. Unrelated to pregnancy and birth, the print derives from a stele in Beijing that was typically used to help Daoist adepts in their processes of bio-cultivation. I had a large copy of the print on my wall in 2008 when I was pregnant with my son and writing my dissertation, the topic of which pertained to art and religion of medieval China. During my pregnancy, I would look at this image every day. Kieran's birth was arduous for many reasons, the most relevant to the discussion of this chapter having to do with my birthing phase of him, which lasted 4.5 hours. About two hours into that process, a registered nurse determined that Kieran was in a posterior position, and I was then able to turn him by rolling back and forth on the bed. But even after he turned, and although I was unmedicated, I was still having difficulty birthing him. Although all monitoring suggested that both the baby and I were fine, I endured numerous suggestions by the medical staff that interventions were necessary. Resisting those suggestions, I at one point remembered the Daoist print from my dissertation and appropriated its imagery, meditating deeply on the mental construct of a large river flowing through my body with a baby riding it and gushing out through its mouth. Shortly thereafter, Kieran was born, weighing in at 9lbs 12oz and 23 inches long. The image has since become sacred to me, although its sacredness relates to the process of birth and not specifically to the practice of Daoism. Although I could not be certain at the time that my personal

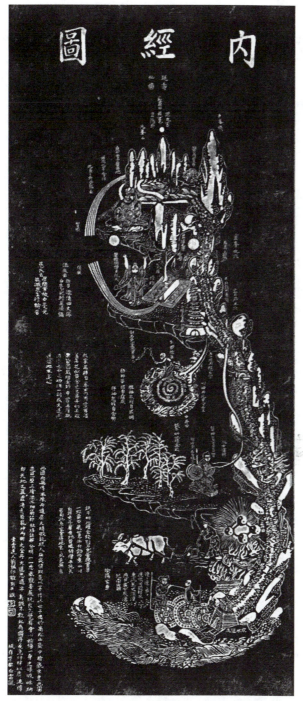

FIGURE 3.1 *Neijing tu* (Diagram of Internal Pathways), Rubbing of Stele, White Cloud Abbey, Beijing, China (photograph Antoni Batchelli)

visualization of the river had led to the way that my son emerged during birth, I was intrigued and thus began my study of images, the visualization of birth, and the sacralization of images used in birth as a rite of passage.

The topics of gestating and being born, as well as those of being pregnant and giving birth, involve complex queries that branch into all areas of philosophy. Yet while canonical philosophers have historically focused on universals in the human experience, including the universal of death, they have given much less attention to birth. This same underrepresentation of the birth topic persists in other areas of the humanities, as well as in the arts. This chapter looks at one particular juncture of philosophy, religion, and art as they converge around the topic of birth. The point of convergence occurs during contemporary rituals of birth, when the ontology of art and material culture about birth alternates between sacred, secular, and re-sacralized spaces. "Ontology" in this context refers to the "being" of the objects, but in their social sense – their social meaning. In preparation for labour and birth, as well as during childbirth itself, pregnant women across cultures are using a diverse range of images to support them and provide mental and physical safety during birth as a rite of passage. An understanding of childbirth as a sacred or spiritual act, often of a nonreligious or humanistic nature, permeates these rituals of birth, and material culture is an integral part of these rituals. Religious objects and rituals involve beliefs and practices related to a superhuman reality, and they are also sacred in the Durkheimian sense of separation from the profane or mundane world. But in many cases, the realm of the nonreligious, often the case in contemporary birth rituals, is also rich with sacred rites and objects. The chapter also takes into consideration artistic treatments of infertility, medical intervention, and menopause, demonstrating that representation of these topics is also part of birth's spiritual dimension.

Childbirth and artistic representation

American artist Judy Chicago embarked on a five-year long project called the "Birth Project" in the 1980s precisely because she was unable to locate images of birth when looking for them. Chicago explains the situation quite well in her 1985 book on the project:

> When I approached this subject matter again in preparation for the Birth Project, I went to the library to see what images of birth I could find. I was struck dumb when my research turned up almost none. It was obvious that birth was a universal human experience and one that is central to women's lives. Why were there no images? Attracted to this void, I plunged into the subject.
>
> *(Chicago 1985, 6)*[1]

Chicago's project comprised a series of monumental needlepoint tapestries depicting birth, created with the help of 130 needleworkers (e.g. see Figure 3.2).

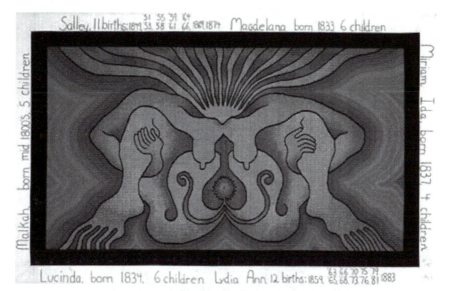

Salley, 11 births: 1871 51 55 59 64, 88 1874 Magdelana born 1833 6 children

Malkah born mid 1800s, 5 children

Miriam Ida born 1837 4 children

Lucinda born 1834 6 children Lydia Ann 12 births: 1859 63 66 70 75 79 65 68 73 76 81 1883

FIGURE 3.2 *The Crowning*, Needlepoint 4, 1984. Needlepoint over painting on mesh canvas, 40 ½" × 61". Painting on canvas by Judy Chicago with Linda Healy; © 1984 Judy Chicago / Artists Rights Society (ARS), New York

As successful as the exhibition tour was, however, Chicago's images of childbirth are abstract and do not show the visceral, realistic aspects of birth.

Jonathan Waller, a contemporary British artist, created just such realistic images, which were shown very briefly in his exhibition, *Birth*, at the Flowers East gallery in 1997 in London. Devoted entirely to paintings of his wife giving birth to their first child, the exhibition withdrew some of Waller's work based on the reaction of viewers who found it offensive. "Is Birth the last taboo subject in art?" wrote Keren David and Mark Rowe, two reporters for *The Independent* who covered Waller's show; "The response to Jonathan Waller's paintings inspired by the arrival of his daughter suggest that it may be. One picture of a woman giving birth was considered so shocking by the staff of a London gallery that it was removed from an exhibition on its opening day."[2] Through his representations (Figure 3.3), Waller had crossed a line and transgressed a taboo. Even today, few images of his paintings exist online, though his catalogues include many works that are important not only to those interested in childbirth but in an art historical sense. Through mechanisms both active and passive, Waller's paintings may be considered suppressed works.

This situation of how childbirth is represented in art has changed since the turn of the century, however, as a contemporary art movement devoted to images of birth has developed rapidly in the United States and abroad. This movement has gained international presence through online image sharing and networking, and through small exhibitions, including a permanent collection,

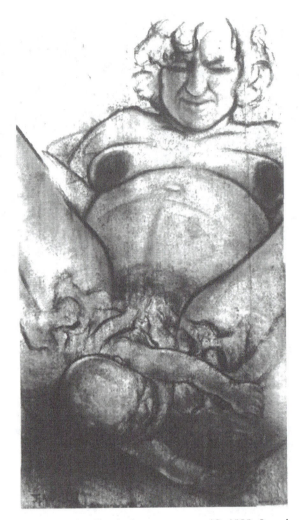

FIGURE 3.3 *Mother No. 58*, oil painting on canvas (© 1998, Jonathan Waller. All rights reserved)

the Birth Rites Collection, which opened in 2008 at Goldsmiths University in London and is permanently located in the Midwifery School of Salford University, Manchester. Since 2010, I have also maintained an extensive online archive of art objects used in birth (visualizingbirth.org). The movement has a wide reach, and its members include artists who create artwork about birth, as well as others interested in using the artwork for personal or professional reasons. Such members are writers, pregnant women, fathers, partners, doulas, midwives, doctors, childbirth educators, yoga instructors, and acupuncturists, among others.[3] Many of those involved are interested in ways to facilitate labour and birth, often with a focus on natural or alternative methods of birth. However, the movement cannot be defined as a natural birth movement since its focus is not on natural birth but on how objects and representations of birth are associated more broadly with birth as an important rite of passage.

This chapter now turns to discussion of a particular way in which some of these objects are used during the contemporary rituals of birth. Of central interest is how the meaning of these objects goes through transformation between the sacred and the secular for people who use them during birth as a rite of passage. In the philosophical sense, this meaning of the object is its *social ontology*, a term that refers broadly to the collective understanding of phenomena that is part of our social world.[4] In the case of birth art and other objects, their ontologies are highly mutable when used during birth, demonstrating how religion, secularity, and sacredness are all interwoven in the contemporary context of birth as a rite of passage.

Religious, secularized, and re-sacralized birth objects

Beginning with religious objects associated with birth and currently used within the birth community, I examine those images that show crowning and other aspects of birth in an overt way. By "birth community," I am here referring to a global phenomenon that includes a broad range of participants in the experience of birth, described earlier and including pregnant women and their partners, members from the medical community, such as midwives, nurses, and doctors, as well as others such as doulas, artists, writers, and educators for whom birth is a central part of their lives. The global nature of this community is clear from the data I present to back up research on the first image of this study, which is that of the Tantric figure (Figure 3.4). As part of the data on that image, for example, I was able to track viewers of the image to a particular website (visualizingbirth.org) as coming from 56 different countries from around the world (six continents: North America, South America, Europe, Asia, Africa, Australia). In looking at all of the other websites that used the image for birth-related purposes, I also noted a diverse range of cultures, a fact represented well in the many different languages used to discuss the image. These languages included Chinese, Danish, Dutch, English, German, Indonesian, Italian, Portuguese, Russian, and Spanish; with one site devoted to nude figures found in Telugu. Appropriated in the context of birth in the twenty-first century, these images are stripped of their religious significations and propagated as simple, secular tools used in labour and birth as a rite of passage.

This image of a divine figure giving birth is a wood carving from India, likely dating to eighteenth century Southern India.[5] Little is known of its precise cultural signification, although popular sources suggest that the figure represented is the Goddess Kali, one of the most important figures in Hinduism. This identification with Kali is erroneous, however. Kali does not have these markings and always has at least two pairs of arms (and usually more).[6] Other sources suggest the figure is an image of feminine divinity found in the contexts of Tantra and Shaktism.[7]

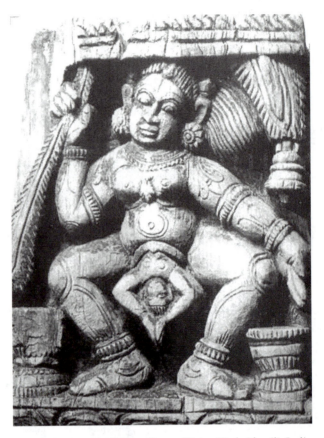

FIGURE 3.4 *Wood Carving of a Divine Figure Giving Birth* (detail) India, eighteenth century. The Mookerjee collection, from *Kali: The Feminine Force* by Ajit Mookerjee. (Thames & Hudson Ltd, London)

In its contemporary online context, however, interest does not focus on the figure as that of a goddess. In fact, almost all of the websites in which she appears have stripped her entirely of religious and cultural identities, providing viewers only with the image of her body. On these websites, which are of a non-religious nature and come from around the world, the image is associated with and promoted for the act that she portrays – that of a woman squatting powerfully to give birth – and information provided on the figure is often minimal or not included at all.

An example of one such website is lotusfertility.com, whose author is Mary Ceallaigh, a certified yoga teacher and midwifery consultant with an academic background in human development. Ceallaigh's page titled "Kali Asana – The Yogic Position for Birth" shows the tantric image alongside photos of actual women squatting in the yogic position. The page goes into significant detail about the benefits of birthing while squatting, but it says nothing about the image itself. The figure is displayed less for its relationship to the divine or sacred than it is for its secular aspects, which show birth positioning and the emergence of a baby.[8] The art image also accentuates the birth process through its unabashed depiction of the vulva, which stretches enormously to facilitate birth. In this contemporary context, the tantric figure helps its viewers on a practical level and not on a sacred one.

Another image with similar purposes is the well-known *Sheela-na-gig*, a stone figure carving identifiable by the figure's large vulva, which opens widely, some say grotesquely, while others claim it to represent the act of birth (Figure 3.5).[9] Originally found in Ireland, Britain and on mainland Europe, the figures, also known simply as "sheelas," measure between 9 and 90 cm and are still present in old churches, churchyards and other fortifications.[10] Scholars generally agree that the figures date from the twelfth to the sixteenth centuries, although some have suggested dating as early as the sixth and seventh centuries.[11] The figures are bald with an upper bony body suggestive of old age.

Much literature describes them as "crones" or "hags." Aside from these features associated with old age, however, the *Sheela-na-gig*'s most distinctive characteristic is its full and enlarged vulva, which is suggestive of vitality and youth. Centered

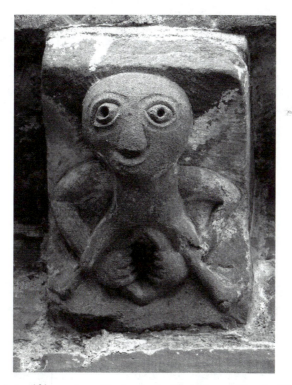

FIGURE 3.5 A twelfth century *Sheela-na-gig*, Church at Kilpeck, Herefordshire, England (© Copyright Zorba the Geek and licensed for reuse under this Creative Commons License)

on the body and typically held open by the sheela's own hands, the vulva is the focal point of the object. The original meaning and purpose of the sheelas remain unknown, and contesting theories as to their origins have circulated since the objects first came to scholarly attention in Ireland during the mid-nineteenth century. Speculation and interest in the figure and its meaning have surged in various disciplines over the past two decades. Some of the most recent works include *Sheela-Na-Gigs: Unravelling an Enigma* (2004) by cultural historian, Barbara Freitag; Maureen Concannon's *The Sacred Whore: Sheela Goddess of the Celts* (2004), developed in the context of history and psychology; Jennifer Regan Borland's iconographic study, *Unstable Women: Transgression and Corporeal Experience in Twelfth-Century Visual Culture*; archaeologist Theresa Oakley's *Lifting the Veil: A New Study of the Sheela-Na-Gigs of Britain and Ireland* (2009); and Georgia Rhoades' *Decoding the Sheela-Na-Gig* (2010), a contribution to women's studies. Although a diverse range of theories has been developed over the years to describe the meaning of the sheela figures, these theories tend to split in three general directions: (1) sheelas represent female divinity and motifs of birth and fertility stemming from pagan understandings of female power; (2) they are connected to Christian warnings against lust and sin as propagated by the medieval Catholic Church; or (3) they are associated with apotropaic devices used within the Church to ward off evil. Within these divisions, scholars have effectively perceived of the *Sheela-na-gig* and its representation of the female body as either sacred, profane, or a combination of the two. In all cases, a common thread emerges to interpret the object's historical meaning: the *Sheela-na-gig*'s ontology is bound to the sacred-profane dichotomy present in modern concepts of religion.[12]

As in the case of the tantric wood carving described earlier, the *Sheela-na-gig* is today used by many who view it as a secular tool to help women during birth. Renowned American midwife, Ina May Gaskin, for example, has written prolifically on the topic of birth for over four decades, and has described the practical utility of the *Sheela-na-gig*:

> My idea is that this figure was probably meant to reassure young women about the capabilities of their bodies in birth. Ellen Predergast, in an article written for an Irish journal, remarked, "After a lifetime's awareness of such figures I am convinced their significance lies in the sphere of fertility, and that is what is depicted … is the act of giving birth." Whether Ms. Predergast and I are right or not, I can testify that a sheela-na-gig figure can be a great help at a birth.
>
> *(Gaskin 2003, 253)*[13]

Gaskin, a highly influential midwife, writer, and proponent of natural birth who has a wide readership and popular presence in the United States and abroad, highlights the object's basic utility as an aid to laboring women. As Gaskin (2003) points out "the vulva of the crouching figure is open enough to accommodate her own head. Such a sight is quite encouraging to a woman in labor" (253).

Although such focus on the *Sheela-na-gig* and others like it appears to revolve around the secular aspects of birth, the utilization of these images in the visualization of birth also takes part ritualistically in birth as a rite of passage; thus, the ritualistic role that these images may play in this rite cannot be ignored. The objects, originally used in contexts associated with religion, are now being transplanted in a trans-religious, transnational and trans-historical way such that they are not only secularized, but are also re-sacralized during contemporary rituals of birth. To understand this process between the sacred and the secular, I now turn to an exploration of ritual in birth as a rite of passage. I contend that the use of images like the two just mentioned plays an integral part in how some women are today preparing ritualistically, as well as practically, for birth.

Ritual and art in birth as a rite of passage

In her comprehensive work on ritual, *Ritual: Perspectives and Dimensions* (1997), Catherine Bell describes birth and birth rituals as providing some of the most foundational models for the ritual processes of most traditional or religious societies.[14] From her theories, it follows that how societies experience birth ritualistically is highly influential in the way that those societies develop other ritualistic traditions. However, in her discussion of secular cultures and the rituals of birth, Bell also states that these societies only mark birth with a few rites. In accord with Bell's thinking here, one finds that birth functions differently or in a lesser capacity as a rite of passage when viewed within its secular context. Yet the secular, claim other scholars, provides rich ground for the rituals of birth. For example, Robbie Davis-Floyd describes in her classic cultural study of birth, *Birth as an American Rite of Passage* (1992), a highly ritualistic nature as inherent in the technocratic model of an American hospital birth.[15] Technological medical procedures in the United States have been standardized in such a way, she maintains, so as to resemble the standardized rituals at the heart of rites of passage attached to birth in traditional societies. In fact, the rituals attached to the secular tradition of a hospital birth have become so elaborate that their complexity surpasses that found in religious societies.[16] As such, the birthing woman within this secular context undergoes a cognitive transformation in which she is socialized through the ritual of birth, incorporated as an individual into a shared belief system whereby she joins others to uphold the authority of the technocratic model of birth in her society.[17] Davis-Floyd also emphasizes the crucial role that symbols play in transmitting the message of the ritual – both to the performers and to the receivers of that ritual.[18] Based on her examination of neurophysiological research, she finds that symbols are not processed intellectually, which typically happens when a message is verbally decoded in the left hemisphere of the brain. Instead, they are *felt* in a totality of body and emotion, often received unconsciously and filtered through the brain's right hemisphere.[19] Davis-Floyd contends that this absorption of symbols is extremely powerful in the shaping of a subject's conformity to the larger social order, giving as an example that of a Marine ordered to sleep with his rifle, repetitively and ritualistically, as a way by which the Marine's superiors reorganize his or her belief patterns to match those of fellow Marines.[20] In this case, the material object of the gun becomes an internalized object and an integral part in how the Marine views his or her way of functioning in the world; namely that the gun and the ability to use it become a part of him or her, almost like an extension of the body.

According to Davis-Floyd, symbols integral to these rituals of birth include everything from a woman's dress in hospital gown and placement in a hospital bed to obstetrical procedures such as electronic monitoring, intravenous feeding, use of pain drugs, epidural analgesia, episiotomies, and cesarean section. Davis-Floyd's focus is on how the rituals surrounding birth in America are frequently of an obstetrical nature, connected to a different and often conflicting rite of passage, which is that of obstetric training. As Davis-Floyd explains, nascent obstetricians are socialized during medical school such that they see birth as a technological event.[21] Within the powerful space of the hospital, she claims, the technocratic model of birth usually replaces the natural model, having the effect of transforming both the rituals attached to the woman's delivery of her baby and to the cognitive and emotional transformations that the woman undergoes during her rite of passage. These transformations occur when the woman's own belief system has the capacity to change.

Paralleling Davis-Floyd's work on the secular ritual of birth as it occurs in the hospital setting is the influential research of Melissa Cheyney, a professor, medical anthropologist, and midwife, who has examined the rituals of birth as they occur in the case of women who birth their babies at home.[22] Cheyney's primary focus is on how these women use rituals to develop ideals about birth that differ significantly from the dominant societal ideologies of birth. She describes the way in which rituals that are part of the natural birth model act to transform women during birth as such:

> As the structure and content of ritual carries participants into new representational spaces, the physical body is transformed along with the participant's social status and sense of self. The performance of birth at home enables women to map their own individual experiences onto a collective, mythic, world – in this case, the mythic world of "natural," "alternative," "empowered," or "woman-centered" childbirth. Emotionally charged symbols (birth tubs, home and reinterpreted technologies like the Doppler) allow social worlds to be manipulated, and it is this manipulation that facilitates a corresponding transformation of the mother's embodied, birthing experience.
>
> *(Cheyney 2011, 535–536)*[23]

The research of Davis-Floyd and Cheyney underscores how material objects involved in birth become emotionally charged and ritualistically meaningful to women before and after their pregnancies. Expanding on this assessment, I propose that religious art and other objects associated with birth have the capacity to become sacred of their own accord, even when secularized and detached from their original religious contexts. These material objects play a part in revering birth as a sacred or spiritual event, and it is in this reverence for birth, and for mothering as well, that the secularized image becomes re-sacralized and treated as a devotional object to be used in birth as a sacred rite of passage.

The role that the object plays here opens up a philosophical discussion related to the extent to which objects as a whole may function on an ideological level between the sacred and the secular; for the objects' users negotiate between these two spheres (the sacred and the secular) in three stages; in the first, the object is sacred and religious; in the second, the object is transformed into a secular and practical tool; and in the third, the object is re-sacralized, becoming sacred primarily in its ritualistic function as attached to birth as a rite of passage. Although the material of the object remains unchanged, its ideological import and social ontology shift between these stages. In their contemporary context, objects such as the *Sheela-na-gig* and the wooden carving of tantric origins are used in birth as a rite of passage, and through the process of the rite, they become sacred in a new way, transformed by their users. In the case of the *Sheela-na-gig,* for example, artisans today have created re-sacralized forms of the object, making an array of sacred charms and pendants of the figure to purchase and use for birth and fertility.

Another similar case in which one clearly notes the secularization and subsequent re-sacralization of objects is that of the birth altar. The birth altar is a sacred place in the home, usually on a table or in a corner that some pregnant women (sometimes with her partner and/or children) creates as she prepares for labour and birth. Objects such as pictures and sculptures related to birth and mothering, written birth affirmations, candles, and ultrasound photos may all be a part of the altar. An altar is itself a religious structure, and objects included on the birth altar also sometimes include religious objects and images, such as those of the Virgin Mary or the Buddha. However, in the context of birth, the altar is usually not a *religious* altar, but instead a spiritual place for the woman and her family as they prepare for birth. A picture of the Virgin Mary may be revered not for its religious content, but because the Virgin is a universal symbol of a woman who gave birth. An understanding of this re-sacralization process of the religious object can be seen, for example, in this parenting website's article on how to construct a birth altar, here as it pertains to the Virgin Mary:

> Look at images of beauty and motherhood. Whether it's a painting of a mother, Mary with Baby Jesus, or whatever you want, find something that seems like a beautiful depiction of the process of bringing life into the world
> *(Haskell 2010)*[24]

A collective understanding of birth as a powerful human event has the power to bring about a transformation of the object's social ontology, taking its meaning from religious and secular spaces to a re-sacralized or newly sacred space.

Turning to an examination of contemporary art related to birth and mothering, I now examine how artists are representing these events as divine or spiritual acts in themselves, inviting their viewers to enter the work with an understanding that the events depicted are sacred. In these works, the sacred and the secular merge, creating a new visual form of sacred secularity in art.

Using acrylic on a large 5' × 5' hand built canvas, Sara Star completed her monumental work, *The Crowning* (Figure 3.6), which depicts the Virgin Mary giving birth to Baby Jesus. While preparing her subject matter, Star researched the topic of Mary giving birth extensively, but she found no images in all of art history that depicted the event.[25] At the time that she was painting the piece, Star was also unable to find any other paintings of natural birth and so referred to photos in a birthing manual. She then studied traditional iconography with a focus on the style of strokes, verdaccio underpainting, and gold leaf halos, ultimately using modern archival materials. She also completed her *Study for The Crowning* (Figure 3.7) before embarking on her painting of the final piece.[26]

In Star's image of the Virgin Mary, the figures shown are sacred, and yet the focus of the painting is on "the crowning," the act of birth itself, which is shared by Mary and Jesus as mother and child. Whereas this is the only image I know of that depicts the actual birth of Jesus Christ, the emphasis in the birth scene is on the humanistic act of birth – an event shared by women and children across time, culture, and history. By focusing on *crowning* and not on the Virgin, Star's painting

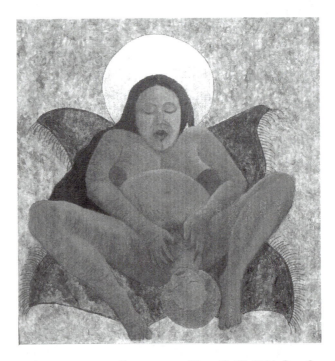

FIGURE 3.6 *The Crowning*, acrylic on canvas (5' × 5') (© 2004, Sara Star. All rights reserved)

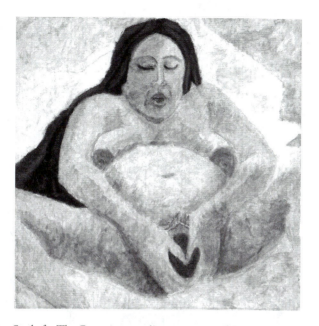

FIGURE 3.7 *Study for The Crowning*, acrylic on canvas (3'×3') (© 2004, Sara Star. All rights reserved)

provides for a powerful inversion of art's historical representations of Jesus and the Virgin Mary. Canonical depictions often represent the Virgin as a mythical symbol of motherhood, which some art historians have described as problematically related to a "patriarchal motherhood" or a "sacrificial motherhood."[27] The word "crowning" also frequently relates to a king, or "the King" in a case such as that of Jesus Christ. As opposed to emphasizing the Virgin as an archetypal, sacrificial, or divine mother, or to referring to a king, however, Star highlights the Virgin's characteristics as a human, a woman, and a mother.

Sacredness is similarly present in Canadian artist Kate Hansen's *Tiara and Eve Marie*, which is part of Hansen's *Madonna and Child* series (Figure 3.8). As with other paintings in this series, Hansen depicts a mother and her baby as adorned by the sacred symbol of the halo. Here, the simple union between mother and child, as opposed to between two religious figures, is that which represents the sacred.

In Star's and Hansen's paintings, religious imagery is not extracted in order to provide viewers with a practical tool used in birth and labour, or to re-sacralize a secularized image. Instead, the artists have depicted birth and motherhood as sacred events that embody transcendental and immanent qualities. And for many women who from around the world examine these images as they prepare for birth, the objects also partake in birth as a rite of passage.

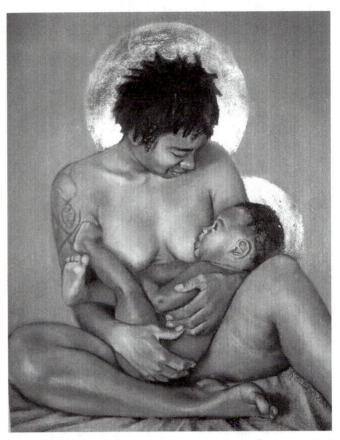

FIGURE 3.8 *Tiara and Eve Marie*, conte crayon and gold leaf on paper (© 2011, Kate Hansen. All rights reserved)

Representation of the marginalized in a discussion of childbirth

In addition to these images of birth and mothering, some members of the same community are also using art and writing to acknowledge other important aspects associated with childbirth and the female body, including infertility, menopause, and medical intervention. Sara Star, the artist just discussed, cannot have children herself and is also working on themes of loss and infertility. She explains the spiritual way in which her paintings, including those about birth, are also a part of this aspect of her life:

> Whenever I have felt down, I remember that actually *The Crowning* and other paintings I make are my babies and they live a life in the world as rich and meaningful as the best child could.

(Star 2016)[28]

For Star, the paintings themselves, as well as the process of making them, is a part of healing. Another American artist who believes in the use of art for personal healing and transformation after trauma is Arla Patch. Patch has worked for decades as a social activist, utilizing art to help groups such as incarcerated women, at risk teens, adolescent male addicts and alcoholics, and women with breast cancer.[29] Some of her artwork is devoted to the topic of spirituality and the female body (see *Godbody*, Figure 3.9), including themes of birth and fertility, and she has even illustrated a coloring book for women trying to conceive.[30] Patch has also created exquisite pieces connected to the theme of menopause. In her relief work, *Homage to the Uterus, Portal of the Uterus* (Figure 3.10) for example, Patch uses coloured coils of clay to reveal an image of two uteruses and their ovaries. While the work on the one hand celebrates the capacities of the uterus, its primary purpose is to express the mourning that some women go through at the end of their childbearing years (others indeed may welcome this transformation). Two white teardrops appear in the image's lower uterus, offering a visual marker of this mourning process. This moment of menopause, characterized by an array of emotions, including sadness, also marks an essential and often sacred rite of passage for a woman as she commences the autumn of her life.

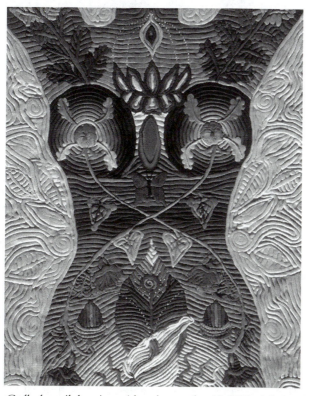

FIGURE 3.9 *Godbody*, coil drawing with polymer clay (© 2012, Arla Patch. All rights reserved)

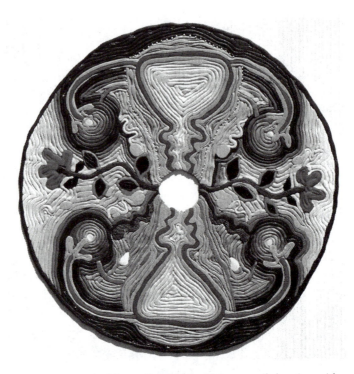

FIGURE 3.10 *Homage to the Uterus, Portal of the Universe*, coil drawing with polymer clay (© 2011, Arla Patch. All rights reserved)

Patch explains some of the complexity of the feelings that may arise during menopause:

> Now as my ovaries are turning away from their full time function of producing eggs and my childbearing ends, I have even greater appreciation for this magnificent, yet hidden part of my body. It was the first home for my son, giving him the start that would make the blueprint for his lifetime.
>
> *(Patch 2011)*[31]

Menopause is a physiological phase that all women will undergo once they pass their childbearing years. As such, this time of transformation is deserving of material representation, and Patch's work offers others the chance to reflect both on the moment and the complexity of its associated emotions.

Jody Coughlin is another artist who creates vibrant images of the pregnant body, usually through watercolor (Figure 3.11). However, she has also written poignantly about her own experiences as a mother who gave birth to her three children through cesarean section, and some of her art addresses the theme of medical intervention. In her writing, Coughlin describes how she on the one hand felt deeply dismayed at the lack of information available to her before giving

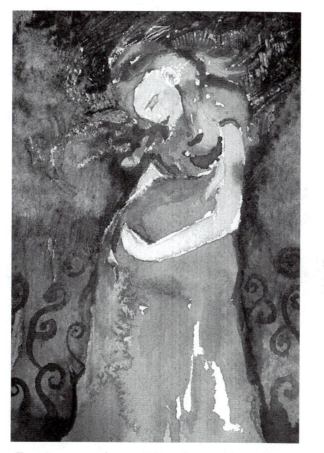

FIGURE 3.11   *Expecting*, watercolor (© 2008, Jody Coughlin. All rights reserved)

birth and leading to the first cesarean when she was only twenty-three years old, while simultaneously feeling ashamed and in need of love and respect from others in the birth community. She writes of how beautiful her baby was to her when she first saw him, a boy of 9lbs 12oz, while also describing the searing pain of the cesarean, and her blurry vision from the pain medications she was given, which she notes must also have been floating through her son's system.[32] All of these conflicting feelings of love, pain, sadness, connection, and separation, are beautifully rendered in Coughlin's painting, *Incision* (see Figure 3.12).

Coughlin's work gives material voice and expression to these sentiments, connecting with others who feel conflicted about the medical interventions they underwent during the process of birth. Although the trauma of the caesarean is clear from the work, the shower of red hearts, a deep symbol of love, bonds mother and baby together, gesturing growth through her challenges of the birthing process. The fragmented quality of the work's colors resembles stained glass through which light streams forth.

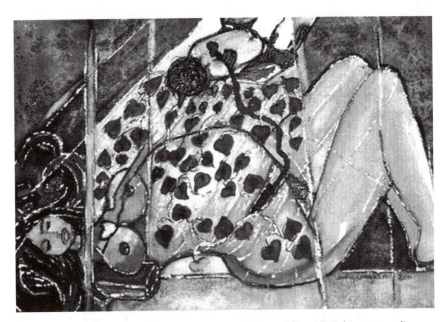

FIGURE 3.12 *Incision*, watercolor (© 2011, Jody Coughlin. All rights reserved)

The arts and humanities: towards a philosophy of birth

This chapter has explored the presence of religious, secular, and re-sacralized art imagery both in the visualization of labour and birth, and as a ritualistic part of birth as a rite of passage. The way that these objects are used points to an important threefold dialectic at play between the sacred and the secular, whereby the secular art object becomes re-sacralized to partake ritualistically in birth. In the ultimate stage of this dialectic, the events of birth and mothering are represented as spiritual acts in themselves, and the viewer therefore enters the artwork right away with an understanding that these events are in fact sacred events. Spirituality is also present in artwork pertaining to topics that are sometimes marginalized in discussions related to birth, including infertility, medical intervention, and menopause.

This chapter reveals how philosophy, religion, and art converge in the context of birth, exemplifing how childbirth, the foundation from which the human experience evolves, is also an event of intellectual and philosophical fascination. One would think that childbirth would be of central interest to the academic sphere of the humanities, and perhaps especially to philosophy. The *humanities*, after all, study the human condition, which is something that begins at birth. But an intellectual underrepresentation of the birth topic persists in the academic world, and this becomes abundantly clear when one compares the academic treatment of birth to that of death. A greater interest in childbirth within the arts and humanities is part of changing our collective understandings of how birth is important not only to women and to children but to philosophy, society, and culture as a whole. Healthcare workers and others working with mothers, families, and babies through childbirth also utilize sacred art and objects, including sacred spaces in birthing centers and birthing rooms, belly casting, and artwork on walls in hospital maternity units. All of these material spaces and representations are an integral part of how birth as a contemporary rite of passage can be celebrated as a sacred event.

Notes

1 Judy Chicago, *The Birth Project*, Garden City, New York: Doubleday & Company, Inc., 1985, 6.
2 Keren David and Mark Rowe, "Birth Paintings Get a Queasy Reception: An Artist's Attempt to Capture the Moment of Childbirth Proved Too Strong for Gallery Staff," *The Independent*, 6 July 1997.
3 I utilize online data sources such as Google Analytics connected to my website to demonstrate the traceability of the movement as a worldwide phenomenon, and I also look at the types of audiences that some of the websites utilizing the images are geared to (see footnote 9 for method and results).
4 For founding ideas on social ontology, see John Searle, *The Construction of Social Reality*, New York: The Free Press, 1995.
5 The image is now part of an extensive art collection begun by the late Bengali scholar of tantric art, Ajit Mookerjee (1915–1990). Ajit Mookerjee, *Kali, The Feminine Force*, London: Thames and Hudson Ltd., 1988, 44.
6 14 February 2013 email communication with Professor David Gordon White, specialist of South Asian religions.
7 In his work, Mookerjee lists the image as, "human birth symbolizing the universal phase of creation. South India, c. 18th century, wood," and the placement of the image occurs in a section of Mookerjee's book devoted to representations of feminine power as found in Tantra and Saktism (Mookerjee, Chapter 2 "Feminine Divinity" [1988], 25–48).
8 Based on the research discussed in footnotes 7 and 8, I cannot say with any certainty that the emerging form is supposed to represent an actual baby or a symbolic one. But for all intents and purposes in terms of its secular usage, it resembles a baby being born in a fantastical way.
9 The term *Sheela-na-gig* is the anglicized form of the Irish term *Sigla na géioch*, which is often translated as "Sheela of the Breasts." For a detailed discussion of the problem of meaning in the name, "Sheela-na-gig," including alternative meanings, see Barbara Freitag's, *Sheela-Na-Gigs: Unravelling an Enigma*, London and New York: Routledge, 2004, 52–67; or Georgia Rhoades, "Decoding the Sheela-na-gig," *Feminist Formations* 22 (2): 167–194.
10 The majority of extant figures are in Ireland, which contains at least 110, with approximately 40 others in England and a handful more in Scotland, Wales, Denmark, Germany and France (Freitag, 3–4).
11 Jack Roberts and Joanne McMahon, authors of *An Illustrated Map of the Sheela-na-Gigs of Britain and Ireland* (1997), believe some of the sheelas date back to as early as the sixth century CE, and early twentieth-century folklorist, Edith Guest, also suggests dates as early as the seventh century CE (Rhoades 167–168).
12 This basic division between the sacred and profane stems from Emile Durkheim's discussion of the dichotomy in his *Elementary Forms of Religious Life* (1912).
13 Ina May Gaskin, *Ina May's Guide to Childbirth*, New York: Bantam Books, 2003, 253.

14 Catherine Bell, *Ritual: Perspectives and Dimensions*, New York, Oxford: Oxford University Press, 1997, 95.
15 Robbie Davis-Floyd, *Birth as an American Rite of Passage*, Berkeley, CA; London: University of California Press, 1992. Religious Studies scholar Pamela E. Klassen has also written extensively on the religious and spiritual aspects of birth in *Blessed Events, Religion and Home Birth in America*, Princeton, NJ: Princeton University Press, 2001.
16 Davis-Floyd 1–2.
17 Ibid. 2–7.
18 Ibid. 9–10. Davis-Floyd's ideas here agree with the symbolic anthropology of Clifford Geertz (this comes from Geertz's, *The Interpretation of Culture*, New York: Basic Books, 1973).
19 Ibid. 9.
20 Ibid. 20.
21 Robbie Davis-Floyd, "Obstetric Training as a Rite of Passage" in *Obstetrics in the United States: Women, Physician, and Society – Special Issue of the Medical Anthropology Quarterly*, 1(3): 288–318, 1987.
22 See: Melissa Cheyney, "Reinscribing the Birthing Body: Homebirth as Ritual Performance" in the *Medical Anthropology Quarterly*, 25 (4): 519–542.
23 Ibid. 535–536.
24 Christie Haskell, "Birth Altar Keeps You Calm Unless You Think It's Weird." 27 December 2010. http://thestir.cafemom.com/pregnancy/113808/birth_altar_keeps_ you_calm
25 Sara Star, personal website: http://sara-star-studio.blogspot.com/2010/11/ responding-to-criticism.html.
26 Correspondence with Sara Star, January 2012.
27 Rachel Epp Buller discusses this issue in the introduction to her volume, *Reconciling Art and Mothering,* Surrey, England and Burlington, VT: Ashgate, 2012, 1.
28 29 August 2016 email correspondence with Sara Star.
29 Patch has been particularly recognized for her projects as a community engagement coordinator working with the Wabanaki people, the Native American tribes of Maine in New England.
30 Buffy Trupp, MA and Arla Patch, MFA, *Coloring Conception: Stress Reduction for Fertility Success,* Vancouver, Canada: The Mindful Fertility Project, 2016.
31 3 December 2011 Correspondence with Arla Patch.
32 Jody Noelle Coughlin, "Why Birth Art" http://poedypencilprincess.blogspot. com/2011/02/why-birth-art.html, accessed 2 September 2011.

References

Bell, C. 1997. *Ritual: Perspectives and Dimensions*. New York and Oxford: Oxford University Press.
Ceallaigh, M. "Kali Asana: Squatting for Childbirth," lotusfertility.com. Accessed 6 January 2011.
Cheyney, M. 2011."Reinscribing the Birthing Body: Homebirth as Ritual Rerformance." *Medical Anthropology Quarterly* 25 (2011): 519–542.
Chicago, J. 1985. *The Birth Project*. Garden City, NY: Doubleday and Company, Inc.
Coughlin, J.N. "Why Birth Art?" http://poedypencilprincess.blogspot.com/2011/02/ why-birth-art.html. Accessed 2 September 2011.
David, K. and Rowe, M. "Birth Paintings Get a Queasy Reception: An artist's Attempt to Capture the Moment of Childbirth Proved Too Strong for Gallery Staff." *The Independent*, 6 July 1997. Accessed June 22 2015. http://www.independent.co.uk/news/ birth-paintings-get-a-queasy-reception-1249258.html.

Davis-Floyd, R. 1992. *Birth as an American Rite of Passage*. Berkeley, CA; London: University of California Press.

Durkheim, E. 1912. *Elementary Forms of Religious Life*. New York: Free Press.

Epp Buller, R. 2012. *Reconciling Art and Mothering*. Surrey, England and Burlington, VT: Ashgate.

Freitag, B. 2004. *Sheela-na-gigs: Unraveling an Enigma*. London and New York: Routledge.

Gaskin, I. M. 2003. *Ina May's Guide to Childbirth*. New York: Bantam Books.

Geertz, C. 1973. *The Interpretation of Culture*. New York: Basic Books.

Haskell C. "Birth Altar Keeps You Calm Unless You Think It's Weird." http://thestir.cafemom.com/pregnancy/113808/birth_altar_keeps_you_calm. Accessed 20 September 2016.

Klassen, P. 2001. *Blessed Events, Religion and Home Birth in America*. Princeton, NJ: Princeton University Press.

Mookerjee, A. 1988. *Kali: The Feminine Force*. London: Thames and Hudson Ltd.

Patch, A. Email communication. 3 December 2011.

Rhoades, G. 2010. "Decoding the Sheela-na-gig." *Feminist Formations* 22 (2): 167–194.

Roberts, J. and McMahon, J. 1997. *An Illustrated Map of the Sheela-na-gigs of Britain and Ireland*. Cork: Mercier Press.

Searle, J. R. 1995. *The Construction of Social Reality*. New York: The Free Press.

Star, S. Email communications. 1 December 2012; 29 August 2016.

Star, S. *The Crowning*. Sara Star Website http://sara-star-studio.blogspot.com/2010/11/responding-to-criticism.html. Accessed 20 September 2016.

Trupp, B. and Patch, A. 2016. *Coloring Conception: Stress Reduction for Fertility Success*. Vancouver, Canada: The Mindful Fertility Project.

White, D. Email communication. 14 February 2013.

PART II

Spirituality and the childbirth year

4

PREGNANCY AND THE UNBORN CHILD

Jenny Hall

Human pregnancy is a powerful and strange time. A human being (or more than one) is developing inside a human being. It is a place of transformation for both the woman and the unborn baby. It is a place, too, of the transformation ultimately into a family, with a change in community and society. The International Confederation of Midwives (ICM 2014) recognises this 'profound experience' that brings 'meaning to the woman, her family and the community' within their philosophy. The aim of this chapter is to focus attention onto the unborn child. As a long-term midwife and mother my consideration of the status of the unborn baby as a human being has evolved, including their spiritual nature within the context of a holistic approach to healthcare.

A mother's story

What does it feel like, being pregnant? I knew. I knew as, I felt different. Not just physical things. This was before the 'missing the period' thing, before the strange metallic taste in my mouth that put me off drinking tea. I knew before the feeling nauseous in the mornings and slightly light headed in the evenings. I knew before I had desperate cravings to eat certain foods such as yoghurt, and very spicy curry, and celery. I knew before the urgency to get to the toilet to empty my bladder. I knew before the stretching of my skin over my lower abdomen. I knew that there was a person inside me. As the weeks moved on that person would become more real, as she moved and shifted in response to the daily moments of my life. Eating meals would provide a variety of responses. Sitting and lying down would be the times of greatest movements and connections between us: they were the times when I was most aware and wanting to connect, sometimes communicating without words, sometimes talking to her. Music playing would either sooth or encourage movements. The effect of this was noted following birth when the music of a favourite soap I had watched during pregnancy would quiet a fractious baby. She is a person now and was a person then inside me. Coming to birth, and shifting from the world of the womb, to the one outside it, we recognised each other, bonded from the relationship we had already developed over the nine months previously. We had some shared genes and a shared experience of motherhood. We still have a shared humanity.

The story above is my story; my story that I went through five times. I have often reflected if the experience of 'knowing' that I had was because I was a midwife and therefore had developed a depth of 'consciousness' about my bodily functions more than others. However, my story is also related by other women (Torngren 2012, Hallett 2002, Stockley 1986, Verny & Kelly 1982). Stories are told here of 'knowing' the 'spirit or soul' of the baby either waiting to enter the body at or before conception; experiencing feelings physically of the presence of the 'spirit' entering the woman; connecting and communicating with the baby while in the womb; and, also, feeling the presence of the 'spirit' of the baby leaving the woman prior to pregnancy loss.

Developing understanding of the mother-baby dyad is complex. The presence of another being alive inside the mother is referred to as a 'mysterious union' (Bergum 1989, 53). In personhood terms a woman can exist without a baby. A woman becomes a mother through the existence of the baby, whether it lives or it does not survive. The baby, in pregnancy, however, is not able to exist in the early weeks or months without the woman/mother host. Though there is 'creation' of a potential person in methods outside the womb for reproductive implantation such as IVF, there is yet to be developments that enable a baby to 'grow' without the mother. The point where a baby is able to 'exist' without a mother is the point of viability. This week of life is different in different countries. In the UK this time according to law is at 24 weeks gestation. However, improved care at birth means that more babies have been surviving at earlier times. In 2006, 491 babies were born alive between 22 and 23 weeks (Costeloe et al. 2012). Though there have been political moves in the past in the UK to reduce the legal week of viability to 20 weeks, the statistical survival rates are very poor prior to 23 weeks, with 15% survival at 23 weeks and 55% at 24 weeks (Tommy's undated). Over the years in the UK I have seen this point drop in weeks as care outside the womb for preterm babies has improved. This point of viability is also legally and ethically different in different countries and societies. Yet there is agreement that the best place, if possible, is for the baby to remain in the host mother's womb for as long as possible to promote the wellbeing of the baby unless there is risk to the health of the mother (RCOG 2014). This indicates that the mother and baby are inextricably linked.

As indicated in the introduction, I am coming to this writing with a background in midwifery practice that has been grounded in the principles of 'holistic' and 'person-centred care'. According to Greenstreet (2006, 25) holistic care is referred to as 'multi-dimensional' and includes 'physical, psychological, spiritual and social aspects'. The integration of whole person and person-centred care is regarded as spiritual care (Clarke 2013). Internationally such principles also lie in the philosophy of midwifery care which states:

> Midwifery care is holistic and continuous in nature, grounded in an understanding of the social, emotional, cultural, spiritual, psychological and physical experiences of women.
>
> *(ICM 2014, 2)*

Though there has been considerable discussion and research around the other aspects of midwifery care identified here, spirituality remains a feature that is ignored. Avoiding the topic, and the aspects of care required, means that women and their babies are not receiving complete, whole-person care.

The soul of the unborn

Defining spirituality has provided challenge to many researchers, and this book illustrates the complexity. Recent discussion recognises the spiritual nature of all people, and that it is an 'innate human characteristic as essential to the wholeness of being as intellectual, physical and emotional attributes' (de Souza & Watson 2016, 346). Analysis of healthcare research papers from 2002–2013 yielded the conceptual definition of spirituality as

> a way of being in the world in which a person feels a sense of connectedness to self, others, and/or a higher power or nature; a sense of meaning in life; and transcendence beyond self, everyday living, and suffering.
>
> *(Weathers et al. 2016, 96)*

Such a definition is applicable in the maternal sense where women experience a depth of connectedness to their unborn babies, as I illustrated in the earlier story, and find a sense of meaning and purpose through the progress of pregnancy as well as the depth of meanings and transcendence that can occur during the process of labour. If we are to understand the 'innate human characteristic' of the spiritual nature of the child in the womb, then we are referring to the 'spirit' or the 'soul' that is inherent.

In an earlier paper, I discussed the roots of the words 'soul' and 'spirit' (Hall 2006) and highlighted they are from different sources. In humanistic contexts the term 'soul' is rarely used as it is more usually associated with religion. Cobb and Robshaw (1998) indicate that the word 'soul' is associated to an inward depth, self-consciousness and wholeness, while 'spirit' is expressed outwardly in relation to expansiveness, consciousness of a God or other being and holiness. Authors write of the centrality of the soul and spirit to the human being as

> the sphere of our being that is whole and complete and wherein we are most authentically our Self.
>
> *(Burkhardt & Nagai-Jacobson 2002, 10)*

For the unborn baby, who has consciousness and memory and communicates with the mother (Hepper 1996, Mampe et al. 2009), it would be logical to consider this human being as a person with a soul.

The question when this baby has a soul in the context of when life begins is debated intensively in religious and secular terms (Hall 2006). The term 'ensoulment' is used to describe this point when the soul 'enters' the person. The recognition of the beginnings of life and 'personhood' of the baby is different according to moral, ethical and legal standpoints (Shaw 2014). The standpoints have also evolved over history through the impact of our understandings of the physical development of the pregnancy and the child, as well as the values in society. The ancient Greek philosophers Hippocrates, Plato and Aristotle began work on understanding the physical development of the embryo, and recognised the concept of the 'soul' (Jones 2004). Early writers from a Christian belief perspective, including Basil the Great, St. Augustine and Thomas Aquinas, debated the principles and did not agree over the timing of ensoulment (Jones 2004). In the Jewish religion ethics in medicine is still impacted by the physician and philosopher Moses Maimonides who wrote in the twelfth century about placing women's needs above those of the unborn (Dunn 1998). The Jewish and Christian discussion is based on the ancient Hebrew Scriptures where beliefs lie of conception as being the point where a pre-existing soul enters the unborn and God is then responsible for 'breathing in the spirit' and the subsequent physical development of the unborn. Within Islamic belief there remains considerable debate as to whether ensoulment is at the moment of conception or at the time of 40 days (Ghaly 2012). The suggestion from the debate is there are three stages of the start of life: conception, gaining 'dignity' at implantation (*ihtiram*) and then achievement of sanctity at the point of breathing the soul at 40 days (*hurma*). Table 4.1 illustrates some of the differing viewpoints across some religions.

In some religious beliefs the presence of the soul of the unborn is a result of reincarnation of another who has lived before. For example, in Hindu belief life is a cycle of birth, death and then rebirth with the unborn choosing the family they are born into due to the deeds they have achieved in a previous life (Gatrad et al. 2004, Jayaram undated). Another example is the view of the indigenous peoples of Australia where spirituality is embedded in the significance of the land and where ancestors and 'spirit children' reside.

TABLE 4.1 Religious views of timing of ensoulment (Hall 2006)

Religion	View of timing of ensoulment
Christian	• Depends on denomination: some at conception, some at implantation • Biblical texts suggest that the fetus may have a spirit
Judaism	• Suggests a fetus may not be a person until it is born, though some have stated that the fetus is a potential person and should be treated with value because of this • Belief that a person has a perfect soul when born and the spirit of that fetus was perfect
Islam	• Ensoulment believed to be either at 120 days (17 weeks), 40 days or when there is movement (12th week up to 20+ weeks) though many believe that life begins at conception
Buddhism	• Believe the moment of conception is the beginning of life of a newly embodied individual
Hindu	• The soul and body forming the fetus are thought to be joined together from conception
Sikhism	• Most believe life begins at conception
Paganism	• Generally believe the spirit is present from the moment of conception • Some believe the spirit of the unborn is present in the house before conception • Others believe the spirit enters later in pregnancy

Previously published in Hall J, 2006. Spirituality at the beginning of life *Journal of Clinical Nursing* 15(7):804–10 Used with permission.

Women receive the pregnancy from the spirits and, at around five months pregnant, when she feels the baby move she will take note of the place where she first felt this as this place will then be significant to that child (Mayra 2012, Carman & Carman 2013). Such beliefs have been compounded further where the receipt of regression hypnosis has appeared to return a person to their previous life or to the womb (Verny & Kelly 1982). Recognition of these issues has resulted in an extensive focus through more mystical and so-called 'new age' beliefs to 'communicate' with the unborn spirit (e.g. Hallett 2002, Carman & Carman 2013).

In the 21st century we are now able to 'look inside' the womb through ultrasound and other visualisation techniques that provide the parents-to-be with a window into the person who is their child. These technological advances have led to fundamental debates within religious denominations (Barnhart 1998, Eisenburg 2004, Athar undated). Women who have religious belief will be influenced by the discussions but it should not be assumed that her beliefs match the doctrine. What is evident is that such techniques may now be having an impact on the parents as they are recognising the 'personhood' of the baby much earlier (Ji et al. 2005). In a Swedish study asking women before an ultrasound what their feelings were about the examination, they talked about meeting the baby and wanting to assess their personality as Gun describes:

> [I]t's kind of getting to see something about how … he or she looks like, or sort of getting a hold of the character …
>
> *(Molander et al. 2010, 21)*

Technology has thus found a way of introducing the baby as a person to their parents long before the moment of birth.

Women's beliefs

For a woman (and her partner), the personhood of the baby is powerfully linked with her beliefs of when life is thought to begin. These beliefs will have impacted on her reproductive choices relating to contraception, termination of pregnancy and screening tests offered during the pregnancy (Hall 2001), her choices for her health behaviours in pregnancy (Heidari et al. 2014a,b, Jesse & Reed 2004) as well as her choice of place of birth and relief for pain in labour (Klassen 2001). The range of beliefs of the personhood of the unborn extends from the moment of conception to when the baby is born. In addition, the values placed on their experience of pregnancy and birth may be intense where they see it is a something that is sacred and holy (e.g. Hebblethwaite 1984, Klassen 2001, Wallas LaChance 1991, Gaskin 2002, Crowther 2013).

Stoyles writes that:

> Relational accounts of fetal value allow that pregnancies have whatever meaning and value they are given by the pregnant woman. Thus, relational accounts allow that pregnancy can have little or no positive value and also that pregnancy can have great value.
>
> *(Stoyles 2015, 93)*

The indication here is the importance of the woman's accounts of her beliefs in the value of the unborn to her. The same paper discusses the views of Lindemann (Stoyles 2015, 94) that the value of the foetus/baby is established by the fact that it has the potential of becoming something of 'moral value'. In addition, the woman 'calls a foetus into personhood' through her behaviours. This implies that, in my own story, as I was so aware of the early 'personhood' of the baby inside me I saw the baby as a human being, rather than a bunch of cells evolving inside me. Lindemann continues that women/mothers act as though the unborn is already a child by 'connecting' through singing and talking and preparing a physical space for the baby by preparing a nursery and buying equipment that is required.

As discussed previously the connections between the mother-baby dyad may begin at any time during pregnancy (e.g. RCM 2012, Torngren 2012, Hallett 2002, Hebblethwaite 1984). However, it is not clear whether this connection is an active choice that women make as an acceptance of the changes taking place in their body or whether it is an internal prompting that makes this connection occur. Suggestions have been made that specific dreams the woman experiences during pregnancy are forms of communication from the unborn (Verny & Kelly 1982, Carman & Carman 2013). However, it is evident that some women would find such communication with their baby more difficult, especially if the pregnancy has not been wanted/expected or if they have previously experienced infertility or pregnancy loss. There is a reluctance to 'connect' and 'guard' themselves through fear of the same occurring again (Dann 2014, Cote-Arsenault 2007, Brockington et al. 2006, Lamb 2002, McGeary 1994). Women may therefore actively choose not to connect with the pregnancy until the 'threat' of the loss has disappeared.

Complexity also arises with the consideration of termination of pregnancy in society as a maternal choice or as offered for a known concern about the wellbeing of the woman or her unborn baby. In the initial scenario, the woman may choose to actively disconnect from the unborn baby. Her beliefs about the personhood of the unborn will have been influenced by her societal background as well as any religious belief she may have, as discussed previously, and this will impact on her subsequent decision about continuing a pregnancy. Evidence points to the necessity of appropriate counselling prior to termination to prevent psychological sequelae, which ensures the woman has made the choice without coercion from others (Dresner & Kurzman 2008, Lipp 2009). These women may return to the maternity services in subsequent pregnancies and experience emotional responses as they reconcile the decisions they have previously made with the feelings for the unborn inside them (Hall 1990). For those women who are subsequently offered termination for a known abnormality of the foetus she may have already reached a place of acceptance and communication with the unborn and the decision making will therefore be more complex. There are documented stories of women who choose to continue with the pregnancy, despite diagnosis of serious life-limiting conditions. In both scenarios maternity carers, partners, other family members and friends need to be supportive and aware of the challenging decisions that the women have made.

The discussion here highlights the complexity of recognising the 'personhood' of the unborn in society where there is acceptance of termination in some quarters, yet not in others. Complex debates are taking place in religious contexts that highlight how the principles of the personhood of the unborn 'fits' within religious societies (e.g. Tsomo 1998, Jayaram undated). In respect of the understandings of women of the personhood of the unborn debates should continue of these topics in order to balance the views so that women are empowered to make appropriate choices for themselves.

Spiritual nurture of the unborn

Carolyn Hastie (2008) has written profoundly of the womb itself as a place for spiritual nurture and meaning. She highlights that the wholeness of the woman and a place of reduced stress and anxiety during pregnancy provides the optimum environment for the baby to grow into wholeness. Evidence is growing of the development of physical illness in later life that has its origins in the womb (Ekbom et al. 1990, Lashner et al. 1993, Ekbom et al. 1996, Wakschlag et al. 2002). Health promotion is being used to promote the health and wellbeing of the woman in order to impact on the health of the child. For example, reduction of smoking in pregnancy and aims to reduce excessive weight gain are being targeted to improve the long-term health of the baby.

In addition emotional disorders in children have been related to incidents in the womb (Hastie 2008, Verny & Kelly 1982). The holistic intertwining of body-mind-spirit (the hyphens are used here in order to illustrate the interconnectedness) would mean any physical or emotional damage could also have spiritual impact. The women in Heidari et al.'s (2014a, b) studies who had a religious belief and faith recognised the sacred nature of the maternal responsibility to keep healthy for the sake of the unborn baby's spiritual wellbeing. They would control their diet, who they spent time with in pregnancy and would aim to avoid stressful situations or challenging environments.

Our increasing knowledge of the impact of emotions, health behaviours and stressful situations on the unborn baby's genes increases the need for us to take more seriously mother's needs during pregnancy (Odom & Taylor 2010).

Implications for care in the antenatal period

The discussions in the chapter will have raised questions for the individual reader. Healthcare practitioners are also human beings with cultural and societal upbringings that will have impact on their beliefs around the start of life. I have raised in a previous paper how these beliefs should be suspended in order to meet the needs and appropriately care for the woman. This may be a challenge where the values women hold are outside the usual expectations of the pathways of care for that society. Maternity carers may be thrown into dilemma as they attempt to support women through their choices and being torn by what they view is the 'right' approach to care. The move to more medical approaches to pregnancy has fragmented the holistic perspective and pushed us into realms where the woman is viewed as a vessel who carries the baby as a passenger. Ethical and moral questions arise of who has the greatest value: the value of the woman or the baby and these questions may only be answered through reverting to the law.

Societal moves have also been toward women making choices to defer having babies until later in their life due to work commitments or later relationships. As a result, there is an increase in artificial reproductive therapies to create babies, as some women may have reduced fertility. Questions then arise of the place and values of the unborn in this situation where there may be a sense of creating a 'commodity' potentially as a provision of 'status' for the mother. Balancing the needs and human rights and respect for the woman and her baby are complex issues that require continuing ethical debate.

The recognition of the spiritual value and needs of the unborn leads to questioning of meeting those needs during pregnancy and beyond. In some cultures, there is respect of the unborn as a 'human and deserves our respect as a symbol of future human life' (ESHRE Task force on Ethics and Law 2001). Ethical discussions should therefore continue surrounding any developments of reproductive interventions and how this will impact on future generations (Odent 2002). Women should be able to make choices with knowledge of the potential impact on the wellbeing of herself and of her unborn baby. However, as Carolyn Hastie (2008) has highlighted, there is also a need to prevent anxiety and stress that may be raised due to introducing these topics.

Childbirth is respected and valued in different ways in many cultures (e.g. Kitzinger 2000). It has been highlighted in this chapter that there are differences in cultural and religious beliefs and faith of the parents that impact on their actions, decisions and values. Care during pregnancy therefore should primarily be individualised to a woman's needs and expectations. Encouraging a woman to talk about her beliefs, and understanding of the unborn will help her to gain an understanding and also to encourage development of relationship. A recent study has demonstrated that an unborn baby will respond to the mother's voice or even to her touching her abdomen (Marx & Nagy 2015). When I read this paper, I was reminded how so many pregnant women do touch and stroke their bodies as they see it change and how, perhaps unknowingly, this is receiving a response form their unborn. Intuitive and responsive behaviours toward their unborn baby should be encouraged to enable greater connection.

Implications for care during birth

Pregnancy and birth are part of an extended continuum. What happens during a pregnancy will then impact on the labour and birth and beyond. Other writers will discuss the spiritual care in labour but there is much to consider around the spiritual needs of the unborn during labour. Increasing technological intervention may be having a long-term effect on future generations (Odent 2002). The increasing use of medicines and interventions to begin labour when the unborn is not ready may have long-term effects on the genetics of the baby (Dahlen et al. 2013). From a belief in reincarnation principles birth at the 'wrong time' may have an impact on the future 'karma' of the individual (Jayaram undated). Further, understanding of memory in relation to the unborn means that lack of care or gentle handling during birth may be 'remembered' in some form (Verny & Kelly 1982, Hepper 1996, Renggli 2005). Providing a calm and respectful environment for welcoming a newborn into the birth space will facilitate the relationship to grow between the mother and the baby and prevent trauma that could have an impact in the long term. More needs to be done to enable women to express their faith and practice their cultural beliefs and rituals to welcome the baby in a safe space.

Conclusion

The aim of this chapter has been to consider the value of the unborn baby and discuss their spirituality in the context of holistic values of mind-body-spirit. Discussion has revealed the unborn child in its personhood, soul and spirit. In exploring the philosophies from a variety of global perspectives I have aimed to encourage further debate. As technology is continually advancing around reproductive technologies the spiritual, ethical and moral values that underpin life should not be ignored. I have aimed to bring forward the voice of women in these discussions who see the importance of the sacred place of pregnancy and childbirth, and the depth of the mother-baby connecting relationship. Despite the increasing worldwide move toward technological controls around birth, women and babies honour this sacred event, and we should do the same.

References

Athar, S. (undated) Islamic perspective in medical ethics. Available from: www.islam-usa. com/index.php?option=com_content&view=article&id=348&Itemid=315

Barnhart, M.G. 1998. Buddhism and the morality of abortion. *Journal of Buddhist Ethics* 5:276–297.

Bergum, V. 1989. *Woman to mother: A transformation.* Granby: Bergin & Garvey.

Brockington, I., Macdonald, E. & Wainscott, G. 2006. Anxiety, obsessions and morbid preoccupations in pregnancy and the puerperium. *Archives Women's Mental Health* 9: 253.

Burkhardt, M.A. & Nagai-Jacobson, M.G. 2002. *Spirituality. Living our connectedness.* Albany, NY: Delmar.

Carman, E.M. & Carman, N.J. 2013. *Cosmic cradle, revised edition: Spiritual dimensions of life before birth.* Berkley, CA: North Atlantic Books.

Clarke, J. 2013. *Spiritual care in everyday nursing practice: A new approach.* Basingstoke: Palgrave Macmillan.

Cobb, M. & Robshaw, V. 1998. *The spiritual challenge of health care.* Edinburgh: Churchill Livingstone.

Costeloe, K.L., Hennessy, E.M., Haider, S., Stacey, F., Marlow, N., Draper, E.S. et al. 2012. Short term outcomes after extreme preterm birth in England: Comparison of two birth cohorts in 1995 and 2006 (the EPICure studies). *British Medical Journal* 345: e7976.

Cote-Arsenault, D. 2007. Threat appraisal, coping and emotions across pregnancy subsequent to perinatal loss. *Nursing Research* 56 (2):108–116

Crowther, S. 2013. Sacred space at the moment of birth. *The Practising Midwife* 16 (11):21–23.

Dahlen, H.G., Kennedy, H.P., Anderson, C.M. et al. 2013. The EPIIC hypothesis: Intrapartum effects on the neonatal epigenome and consequent health outcomes. *Medical Hypotheses* 80 (5):656–662. doi:10.1016/j.mehy.2013.01.017.

Dann, L. 2014. *Women's experience of pregnancy and early motherhood following repeated IVF treatment: A phenomenological study.* A thesis submitted in partial fulfilment of the requirements for the degree of Doctor of Health Science. Available from: http://aut.researchgateway.ac.nz/bitstream/handle/10292/7213/DannL.pdf?sequence=3

Dresner, N. & Kurzman, A. 2008. Psychological aspects of abortion. *Global Library of Women's Medicine* (ISSN: 1756-2228). doi:10.3843/GLOWM.10417.

Dunn, P. 1998. Maimonides (1135–1204) and his philosophy of medicine. *Archives of Disease in Childhood* 79: 227F–228F.

Eisenburg, D. 2004. *Abortion in Jewish law.* Available from: www.aish.com/ci/sam/48954946.html

Ekbom, A., Adami, H., Helmick, C.G., Jonzan, A. & Zack, M.M. 1990. Perinatal risk factors for inflammatory bowel disease: A case control study. *American Journal of Epidemiology* 132: 1111–1119.

Ekbom, A., Hsieh, C.C., Lipworth, L., Wolk, A., Ponten, J., Adami, H.O. & Trichopoulos, D. 1996. Perinatal characteristics in relation to incidence of and mortality from prostate cancer. *British Medical Journal* 313: 337–341.

ESHRE Task Force on Ethics and Law 2001. The moral status of the pre-implantation embryo. *Human Reproduction* 16: 1046–1048.

Gaskin, I.M. 2002. *Spiritual Midwifery*, 4th edn. Summertown, TN: Book Publishing Company.

Gatrad, A.R., Ray, M. & Sheikh, A. 2004. Hindu birth customs. *Archives of Disease in Childhood* 89 (12):1094–1097.

Ghaly, M. 2012. The beginning of human life: Islamic bioethical perspectives. *Zygon* 47 (1):175–213.

Greenstreet, W. (ed.) 2006. *Integrating spirituality in health and social care: Perspectives and practical approaches.* Oxford: Radcliffe.

Hall, J. 1990. A hard decision ... termination of an unwanted pregnancy. *Nursing Times,* 86 (47):32–35.

Hall, J. 2001. *Midwifery, Mind & Spirit: Emerging issues of care.* Oxford: Books for Midwives.

Hall, J. 2006. Spirituality at the beginning of life. *Journal of Clinical Nursing* 15 (7):804–810.

Hallett, E. 2002. *Stories of the unborn soul: The mystery and delight of pre-birth communication.* Bloomington, IN: iUniverse.

Hastie, C. 2008. The spiritual and emotional territory of the unborn and newborn baby, in: K. Fahy, M. Foureur, C. Hastie (eds) *Birth territory and midwifery guardianship.* Oxford: Books for Midwives.

Hebblethwaite, M. 1984. *Motherhood and God.* London: Geoffrey Chapman.

Heidari, T., Ziaei, S., Ahmadi, F., Mohammadi, E. & Hall, J. 2014a. Maternal experiences of their unborn child's spiritual care: Patterns of abstinence in Iran. *Journal of Holistic Nursing* 33 (2):146–158.

Heidari, T., Ziaei, S., Ahmadi, F. & Mohammadi, E. 2014b. Powerful leverages and counter-currents in the unborn child spiritual care: A qualitative study. *Global Journal of Health Science* 7 (1):122–132. doi:10.5539/gjhs.v7n1p122.

Hepper, P.G. 1996. Fetal memory: Does it exist? What does it do? *Acta Paediatrica Supplement* 416: 16–20.

International Confederation of Midwives (ICM) 2014. *Philosophy and model of midwifery care* [online]. Available from: www.internationalmidwives.org/assets/uploads/documents/CoreDocuments/CD2005_001%20V2014%20ENG%20Philosophy%20and%20model%20of%20midwifery%20care.pdf

Jayaram, V. (undated). *Hinduism and abortions* [online]. Available from: www.hinduwebsite.com/hinduism/h_abortions.asp

Jesse, D.E. & Reed, P.G. 2004. Effects of spirituality and psychosocial well-being on health risk behaviors in Appalachian pregnant women. *Journal of Obstetric, Gynecologic, & Neonatal Nursing* 33 (6):739–747.

Ji, E.K., Pretorius, D.H., Newton, R., Uyan, K., Hull, A.D., Hollenbach, K. & Nelson, T.R. 2005. Effects of ultrasound on maternal-fetal bonding: A comparison of two- and three-dimensional imaging. *Ultrasound in Obstetrics & Gynecology* 25 (5):473–477.

Jones, D.A. 2004. *The Soul of the Embryo*. London: Continuum.

Kitzinger, S. 2000. *Rediscovering birth*. London: Little, Brown and Co.

Klassen, P.E. 2001. *Blessed events: Religion and home birth in America*. Princeton, NJ: Princeton University Press.

Lamb, E.H. 2002. The impact of previous perinatal loss on subsequent pregnancy and parenting. *The Journal of Perinatal Education* 11 (2):33–40.

Lashner, B.A., Shaheen, N.J., Hanauer, S.B. & Kirschner, B.S. 1993. Passive smoking is associated with an increased risk of developing inflammatory bowel disease in children. *American Journal of Gastroenterology* 88:356–359.

Lipp, A. 2009. Termination of pregnancy: A review of psychological effects on women. *Nursing Times* 105 (1):26–29.

Mampe, B., Friederici, A.D., Christophe, A. & Wermke, K. 2009. Newborns' cry melody is shaped by their native language. *Current Biology* 19:1994–1997.

Marx, V. & Nagy, E. 2015. Fetal behavioural responses to maternal voice and touch. *PLOS one* [online]. Available from: http://journals.plos.org/plosone/article?id=10.1371/journal.pone.0129118

Mayra. 2012. *The dreaming – Australian Aboriginal peoples*. Available from: http://partopelomundo.com/blog/2011/12/30/the-dreaming-australian-aborigenes/

McGeary, K. 1994. The influence of guarding on the developing mother–unborn relationship, in: P.A. Field & P.B. Marck (eds) *Uncertain motherhood: Negotiating the risks of the childbearing* years. London: Sage Publishing.

Molander, E., Alehagen, S. & Berterö, C.M. 2010. Routine ultrasound examination during pregnancy: a world of possibilities. *Midwifery* 26 (1):18–26.

Odent, M. 2002. *The farmer and the obstetrician*. London: Free Association Books.

Odom, L.N. & Taylor, H.S. 2010. Environmental induction of the fetal epigenome. *Expert Review of Obstetrics & Gynecology* 5 (6):657–664.

RCM. 2012. Maternal emotional wellbeing and infant development: A good practice guide for midwives. Available from: www.rcm.org.uk/sites/default/files/Emotional%20Wellbeing_Guide_WEB.pdf

RCOG. 2014. Perinatal management of pregnant women at the threshold of infant viability (the obstetric perspective). Available from: www.rcog.org.uk/globalassets/documents/guidelines/scientific-impact-papers/sip_41.pdf

Renggli, F. 2005. Healing and birth. *Journal of Prenatal and Perinatal Psychology and Health* 19: 303–318.

Shaw, A. 2014. Rituals of infant death: Defining life and Islamic personhood. *Bioethics* 28 (2): 84–95.

de Souza, M. & Watson, J. 2016. Understandings and applications of contemporary spirituality: Analysing the voices, in: M. de Souza, J. Bone & J. Watson (eds) *Spirituality across disciplines: Research and practice*. Switzerland: Springer.

Stockley, S. 1986. Psychic and spiritual aspects of pregnancy, birth and life, in: R. Claxton (ed.) *Birth matters: Issues and alternatives in childbirth*. London: Unwin Books, pp. 79–98.

Stoyles, B.J. 2015. The value of pregnancy and the meaning of pregnancy loss. *Journal of Social Philosophy* 46 (1):91–105.

Tommy's (undated). *Premature birth statistics* [online]. Available from: www.tommys.org/our-organisation/why-we-exist/premature-birth-statistics

Torngren, P. 2012. *Voices from the womb: Four mothers tell about prebirth communication* [online]. Available from: www.parenting-with-love.com/voices-from-the-womb-prebirth-communication/

Tsomo, K.L. 1998. Prolife, prochoice: Buddhism and reproductive ethics feminism & nonviolence studies, Fall [online]. Available from: www.fnsa.org/fall98/tsomo.html

Verny, T. & Kelly, J. 1982. *The secret life of the unborn child*. London: Sphere Books.

Wakschlag, L.S., Pickett, K.E., Cook, E., Jr, Benowitz, N.L. & Leventhal, B.L. 2002. Maternal smoking during pregnancy and severe antisocial behavior in offspring: A review. *American Journal of Public Health* 92: 966–974.

Wallas LaChance, C. 1991. *The way of the mother: The lost journey of the feminine*. London: Vega.

Weathers, E., McCarthy, G. & Coffey, A. 2016. Concept analysis of spirituality: An evolutionary approach. *Nursing Forum* 51 (2):79–96.

5

SPIRITUAL QUESTIONS DURING CHILDBEARING

Ingela Lundgren

In this chapter I will discuss the period from pregnancy to the birth – i.e. childbearing – with a focus on the role of healthcare professionals. I use the concept 'childbearing' since pregnancy and the birth should be seen as a process and in wholeness which is also of importance for continuity of care (Bryar and Sinclair 2011). The focus of this chapter is the role of healthcare professionals when childbearing is seen as something more than a biomedical condition. Practical examples based on research will be discussed using the central concepts partnership, reciprocity and relationship. My research has been mainly carried out in a Swedish maternity care context where midwives are the primary caregivers for women with normal pregnancy and birth. However, the findings can be transferred to, and be relevant to, other contexts where health professionals are involved in the care.

Childbirth and meaning

The focus for my research is the meaning of pregnancy and birth for women's lives. Meaning is individual and can be related to spiritual questions (Crowther and Hall 2015). Spirituality does not require a religious orientation in order to be embraced; it can speak to secular and religious people alike (Pembroke and Pembroke 2008). Other concepts related to meaning are that of existence (Marcel 1956) and a 'border situation' (Jaspers 1963) – concepts rooted philosophy. Existentialism is a tradition focusing on human uniqueness, freedom of choice and responsibility. According to Marcel (1956) being in the world is the sense of presence, the sense of one's own presence and the sense of the presence of things and of something beyond oneself. A border situation is defined as a condition that in some way expresses the contradictions of being, tied to unsolvable problems, to suffering and to developing forces (Jaspers 1963). Jaspers exemplified death, to struggle, suffering and guilt as border situations. My research indicates that birth can be seen as an existential situation influencing the life of women, and as a 'border situation', a situation that both can develop strength and suffering (Lundgren 2004).

My initial research into childbearing is grounded in my experiences as a midwife (Lundgren 2002). When practising midwifery I met women who, in different ways, described giving birth. Some radiated harmony and happiness and told me that the experience had had a great positive influence on them. Simply by looking at them I could see that giving birth had been empowering and strengthening. However, I have also encountered women who told me that giving birth was the worst experience in their life; a terrifying engagement with fear of death, which they hoped they would never experience again. These encounters inspired me to study childbirth experiences and, specifically, the meaning of giving birth for the lives of women. The journey into meaning usually involves self-transcendence (Pembroke and Pembroke 2008). A transformative experience implies victories and strength, healing, and short- and long-term outcomes. This mother provides an example:

> You see things totally different afterwards, you have another way of understanding … you accept things differently, you become stronger, you can cope with things better than before …before petty details could ruin life, and now you just shake it off your shoulders, you don't become another personality … but you mature and become a stronger personality, when you've had a baby and have gone through that pain. I think that is the purpose of it, what the meaning of life is. I think it is to protect our children, to be stronger, a way of managing everyday life and become stronger, and that it is a life from your own flesh and blood and that too helps you to go through the delivery.
>
> *(Lundgren and Dahlberg 1998, 108)*

A traumatic birth experience on the other hand could have a long-lasting effect on the woman's health and well-being as this mother recounts:

> The labor care has hurt deep in my soul and I have no words to describe the hurt. I was treated like a nothing, just someone to get data from.
>
> *(Beck 2004, 32)*

Women's experiences during pregnancy

I will start with three Swedish studies where women described spiritual existential and meaningful experiences during pregnancy. One study is based on diaries written by women during the three trimesters of pregnancy (Lundgren and Wahlberg 1999). The second study is based on interviews with primiparous women (week 10–14) (Modh et al. 2011). The third study is based on drawings made by women in early pregnancy as a starting point for an interview focusing on the pregnant body (Bergbom et al. 2016).

The study based on women's diaries shows that 'transition to the unknown' during pregnancy is central, which includes meeting one's life situation, meeting something inevitable and preparing for the unknown. The 'transition to the unknown' includes travelling from the past, through the present, towards the unknown and the future (Lundgren and Wahlberg 1999). In the first trimester, women's feelings about their life situations and about their relations to people around them are primary. Descriptions about the past may outnumber those of the future (Lundgren and Wahlberg 1999). Early pregnancy is a life-opening for women, including both life affirmation and suffering and a process of opening up to different dimensions of life (Modh et al. 2011), where the body is connected to the cycle of life (Bergbom et al. 2016). The following women narrate how:

> Then there are grander thoughts about, well the whole world and the state of things. Being pregnant feels like an amazing miracle but it also awakens a lot of thoughts. I'm not religious, but it prompts some kind of religious contemplation, about whether there is something greater that controls things, well, I don't know how to explain.
>
> *(Modh et al. 2011, 7)*

> I have a strong power inside me, but it's not my own power, it's something else. I suppose it's the other soul who wants to come down to earth, I think it's the soul of the foetus that I feel.
>
> *(Modh et al. 2011, 7)*

> There is a kind of calmness in my body that I haven't felt before. I feel that I'm in balance with myself thanks to this power.
>
> *(Bergbom et al. 2016, 5)*

In early pregnancy, some women may express themselves as being chosen and refer to a feeling of holiness. For the women, a life-opening leads to being confronted with questions of life and to see certain values from a wider perspective. This is to meet and reflect on their own existential and spiritual values (Modh et al. 2011). These are further descriptions from women during early pregnancy:

> Well, I think quite a lot about my father who is no longer with us, not frightening thoughts, more a sense that life carries on in spite of the fact that he is no longer here and that he is still with me. It feels a bit, when I think about father in such moments, when I think of him very intensely then I get sad that he can't be a part of this. But then again, I know that he will anyhow. Something like that, it feels like I think of him both in a positive and a negative way well ... the grieving is like, it came back in a way now when I became pregnant. I thought a lot about him but then ... back then I could become very sad, as if attacked by grief. Now I think

about it in a more practical way, well that the family will live on now, Mother will have a life again, it will make her happy ... well things like that, I think quite a lot about family.

(Modh et al. 2011, 5)

Compared to the diaries from the second and third trimester, women wrote more about their life histories and the past in early pregnancy. All aspects of their lives were reflected on: themselves, family, friends, economy and earlier pregnancy, abortions and births (Lundgren and Wahlberg 1999). This woman reveals how she is absorbed into her life history:

I needed much time for myself in the beginning, several hours a day to think about myself, my parents, my childhood, and my fiancé, there wasn't time for any intellectual work the first months. I was completely absorbed by my life history and I thought more about the past than the future.

(Lundgren and Wahlberg 1999, 15)

In the second trimester, feelings of encountering a situation outside their personal control dominated. The women also described this period as a time of fewer physical problems and of living in the present without reflections on the past or the future. This woman explains:

Very uncommunicative, enjoying myself and just being. Feeling better and better. I don't think about anything special. Everything is magic.

(Lundgren and Wahlberg 1999, 16)

In the third trimester preparing for the unknown is central for women (Lundgren and Wahlberg 1999). The women expressed ambivalence in their thoughts about the birth including expectations, longing and worry. Some women described how they were ready to give birth, but others described a hesitation of meeting the unknown:

To be pregnant is not so exciting any more. It's mostly hard work. However, a longing for the baby has arisen. I'm longing to be a mother. Holding up, don't want to give birth, regret, afraid, don't dare, afraid of everything physical. Do I really want a baby to come out between my legs?

(Lundgren and Wahlberg 1999, 17)

Experiences of birth from women's and midwives perspectives

The studies above show that the existential dimensions appear to be central for women during pregnancy. This is also central during the birth and implies for women an encounter with herself as well as with the midwife (Lundgren 2002).

After birth the woman feels changes, which are expressed as being both stronger and more vulnerable:

> I see the delivery as a milestone that, in a way, has helped me to grow as a human being, and you don't forget that but this has just made me stronger and more vulnerable too, although I don't know how to explain it … it outweighs the strength you get so if you are more vulnerable you can manage it much better.
>
> *(Lundgren 2004, 350)*

The life-opening that starts during early pregnancy continues during the birth when forces related to both suffering and strength may be developed, which can be explained with the concept of the 'border situation'. When entering the process of childbearing, encounters are important for the woman that are related to stillness and change (Lundgren 2002). Stillness means for the woman being in the moment – exemplified as presence and being in one's body. Change is expressed as transition – to the unknown and to motherhood. For the midwife stillness and change equals being both anchored and a companion. To be a companion is to be an available person that listens to and follows the woman through the process of childbirth. To be anchored is to be the person that, in the birth process, respects the limits of the woman's ability as well as her own professional limits (Lundgren 2002).

Being an *anchored companion* is related to as one's own professional role. These aspects cannot be handed over to other supporting persons around the woman such as the doula and the partner. Other supportive persons have the role of being supportive and coaching the woman and cannot interfere and act in a border situation as the midwife. Giving birth is both a natural process demanding a non-interventionistic approach and a situation that can suddenly demand activity. Being an anchored companion is easier if the midwife knows the woman and understands her unique needs. This is exemplified by one midwife:

> To use the woman's capacity. What they think about. It takes different time for different women, but I think most women can do this if you give them enough support. And afterwards they can say: 'I can do this. Good Lord, what I can do. My body is capable.' You get so aware of your body's capability. I think this is good for the women.
>
> *(Lundgren 2002, 159)*

Being a *companion* means supporting the woman through her individual process during the birth. A trusting relationship is of importance for this process. When the woman is surrendering herself to the process of birth she needs to concentrate and enter her inner self. The experience of time may be different during the birth and women may express how they are in another world. The woman needs to feel secure for letting go and to follow the process of birth, as these women attest:

> It was very important that I felt secure. Then I could listen to my body and wasn´t so frightened. I gained control over the whole plan and it worked
>
> *(Berg et al. 1996, 13)*

> I'm a person that needs control but didn't need that now ... I felt secure and could let go and just be in my inner self and just be secure there.
>
> *(Lundgren 2010a, 177)*

The woman may have a distinct memory of the midwife even if she is 'in another world' as this mother describes:

> What she [the midwife] said got me through, even though I was another level ... it's like a different level of the brain picks it up, and that bit of the brain reassures the rest of the brain that it's all right.
>
> *(Anderson 2000, 121)*

> She [the midwife] left marks forever on my retina.
>
> *(Lundgren et al. 2009, 120)*

It is of importance when preparing for birth during pregnancy that healthcare professionals discuss control with women. Ask women how they experienced control during their previous birth and for primiparous prepare them for this aspect. Control during birth means both going with the flow and taking command of oneself, and placing the control on persons, the environment and techniques outside oneself. The way women handle control during birth differs between women but can also differ for the individual woman during the process of birth (Lundgren 2004). It is important that women feel safe to let go and allow the body to be in control. There is a sense of 'letting go' yet still not losing control. The worst situation is the feeling that nobody has control over the labour and being 'out of control' (Anderson 2000).

Being *anchored* means the midwife steps in when the situation is calling for action. A woman describes how she experienced a situation when there was no possibility of proceeding:

> I had lost focus and it was just continuing and continuing and I had reached all my boundaries, physically as well as mentally, I was just blubbering and wanted to die. I was in a cul-de-sac like having fastened in a hack in a record. I was sort of locked in a cave and I couldn't get through anywhere.
>
> *(Lundgren 2004, 349)*

If the woman is in this situation, needing to surrender to technique, the midwife needs to proceed and take action:

> I can't get through anywhere, I'm totally deadlocked and at this moment of great despair it seemed that a kind of 'laser elevator' came down and that

the doors opened, and 'Welcome! Step inside and you will be delivered' there is a way out.

(Lundgren 2004, 349)

Being an anchored companion involves taking an active role by steering the birth with clear instructions to the woman and distinct eye contact. The midwife needs to 'catch the woman' and help her back to the process of birth, as this mother explains:

> I had too much Entonox [and] totally lost control ... when I had the worst contractions and then she just ... she said that now you have to listen to me and now you have to be more focused and this will make you tougher and this was just what I needed at that moment.
>
> *(Lundgren 2010a, 178)*

One midwife describes how she needed to be authoritarian and communicate more clearly in order to 'seize the woman' back to the process of birth if the woman is near the limit of her capacity. At the same time the midwife needs to have a trusting relationship with the woman. The midwife describes the moment:

> She was almost fainting and I was losing contact with her, and she was breathing very fast. And her eyes were rolling. And then you have to be distinct, you show her that 'I am here and I can help you'. And I must be more authoritarian, and react. I can't just follow her. I can't let her go. It is my duty. I get authoritarian and say, now we do this. But afterwards they have told me that they have experienced me as being very calm.
>
> *(Lundgren and Dahlberg 2002, 161)*

Afterwards the woman in the above birth told the midwife that she experienced good support. A woman after birth can describe how they lose control and experience themselves as being in a 'border situation'. It can be described as being in a black hole, a very painful experience:

> It was sort of a long black hole. It felt like no let up, just endless, endless pain. Nothing to hold on to ... The feeling in my chest of becoming totally empty ... It's that feeling ... drained of strength and energy and zest for life.
>
> *(Nilsson et al. 2012, 304)*

Women with negative or traumatic birth experiences may develop post traumatic stress and fear of childbirth. Women's perception of the overall birth experience as negative seems to be more important for explaining subsequent fear of childbirth than mode of delivery (Nilsson et al. 2010). A negative birth experience remained etched in the women's minds and gave rise to feelings of fear, loneliness, lack of faith in their ability to give birth and diminished trust in maternity care. The women felt as if they had no place there, that they were unable to take their place, and that even if the midwife was present, she did not provide support (Nilsson et al. 2010).

Being an anchored companion may develop emotions in midwives that they need help to handle. Caring can cause emotional suffering in healthcare professionals due to the high degree of empathic identification which place midwives at risk of experiencing secondary trauma (Leinweber and Rowe 2010). Hunter (2009) describes different ways for midwives to manage their emotions depending on context and individual circumstances. Affective neutrality means to suppress the emotions and deal with them outside the work environment. It may serve as self-protection from uncomfortable feelings but may lead to withdrawal, disengagement and leaving the profession. Affective awareness means focusing emotional responsiveness and expressions. Emotions from the woman and her relatives are accepted; it is better to express what one feels than suppress. The midwife needs to get the balance right in relation to emotion management. A 'with-woman' model of care facilitates affective awareness compared to 'with institution' where this aspect is less central.

Partnership, reciprocity and relationship

Care during childbearing in many countries is mainly influenced by the medico-technical approach where medical interventions are the main focus (Downe 2008). Care systems that support normal psycho-social birthing are globally rare, and have been described as 'lighthouses in an ocean of over-medicalized care' (Davis-Floyd et al. 2009, 1). Therefore, existential questions seem to be neglected in maternity care (Bondas and Eriksson 2001). Further, maternity care has moved into a tick-box culture to ensure 'everything is covered including the midwives' back', to prove the care has been completed. In such culture the depth of spirituality that inheres uniquely in the experience of childbirth remains silenced and hidden (Crowther and Hall 2015). In Sweden, as in many other countries, the first visit during pregnancy is carried out mid-pregnancy. Many medical tests and examinations are carried out at this time and there is a tendency to neglect a woman's life-world and focus mainly on medical issues (Olsson 2000). Therefore women may be left lonely during the life-opening in early pregnancy.

Women express a need for meeting health professionals during this period (Modh et al. 2011). It is important that midwives and other health professionals know and ask women about their individual experiences during early pregnancy, including the relationship with their baby(s). Women may describe that the relationship to the child started in pregnancy with individual variance, ranging from a feeling of the child's presence after conception to a feeling of distance from the child during the last week of pregnancy (Lundgren and Wahlberg

1999). This is verified by Bergum (1997) who says that the woman's unique relationship with the baby – being a mother while being herself – starts in pregnancy, as this mother eloquently describes:

> I clearly felt the moment of conception as an intensive generation of heat around the ovaries and the uterus. As if something is happening 'in there' without my assistance. What a fantastic feeling, to give oneself up to something that happens. And then a feeling of dizziness.
>
> *(Lundgren and Wahlberg 1999, 17)*

The transformative experience may be related to the relationship with the child. One woman describes that during pregnancy she hesitated and had not prepared to be a parent. Her birth story involves pain and strength, and 14 days after the birth she felt a changed state of mind:

> It was exciting. I hardly ate or slept. It lasted for two weeks. And my sister told me I was totally speeded when she talked to me by telephone. I'm so happy for having this experience. For us it was really important because we didn't want this child. It meant everything. I have never been so in love in my whole life as I became in him.
>
> *(Lundgren 2010b, 64)*

This can be described as 'peak experience' (Maslow 1979). A 'peak experience' is characterised by joyous and exciting moments in life, involving sudden feelings of intense happiness and well-being, wonder and awe, and also possibly involving an awareness of transcendental unity or knowledge of higher truth (Maslow 1979). Lahood (2007) claims that traditional birth in different cultures is connected to experiences of non-ordinary states of consciousness, such as 'religious' and 'peak'. Many women find strength and wisdom by passing through these states in labour. However, these descriptions of birth disappeared as childbirth became a purely biomedical issue performed in hospital settings.

A strengthening birth has a potential for healing a previous negative birth experience (see Gill Thomson, Chapter 10). One woman described that during her first birth she felt totally alienated from herself and the midwife, without receiving support and having a feeling that the midwife was afraid of her and the birth. After the birth the woman felt fear and was depressed and sad. She described how she had to handle these feelings by trying to find out what was happening during the birth and by receiving professional support from midwives, physicians and psychologists. This is how she describes her next birth:

> I needed help and my husband knew I was afraid. It [the first birth] was awful. I was very sad for a long time after that birth and it was hard for other people to understand. My mother in law and my mother and

everybody thought everything went well and I had a healthy baby. You didn't have to have a caesarean or anything, so you should be pleased. I was really sad, but the last birth healed everything.

(Lundgren 2010b, 64)

Because pregnancy and childbirth cannot be separated it is important for health professionals to ask women during pregnancy about their previous birth experiences. If needed they should refer to other professionals such as physicians and psychologists. A problem in our current medically driven systems of care is a lack of time for questions other than those that are biomedically focused. However, the existential questions should be raised by listening to the woman and meeting her as a unique individual in an open-minded way, as this midwife explains:

The way in which you ask is important; often you have a standard question: When did it start? What is the pain level? etc. But instead, ask her open questions: How has the last day been? Do you feel ready to give birth? What do you think and feel about the childbirth? and so on. And sometimes I think you can meet the woman there and find out things that would not have been expressed otherwise.

(Lundgren and Dahlberg 2002, 157)

Midwifery continuity of care and women-centred care

Through continuity of care the same professionals are responsible for care during both pregnancy and childbirth, which may help in focusing on these existential questions. Midwife-led-care means the midwife is the lead healthcare professional responsible for the planning, organisation and delivery of care given to a woman from the initial booking of antenatal visits to care during the postnatal period (Rooks 1999). The midwife-led model of care is woman-centred and based on the premise that pregnancy and childbirth are normal life events and can be complementary to the medical model. Women receiving midwife-led continuity models of care are less likely to experience intervention and more likely to be satisfied with their care with at least comparable adverse outcomes for them and their infants than women who received other models of care (Sandall et al. 2016). It is therefore a model of care worth striving for globally. Continuity of care also helps facilitate women-centered care. Woman-centred care is a concept describing care that focuses on the woman's perspective (Bryar and Sinclair 2011) and is related to person-centred care (Ekman et al. 2011), patient-centred care and patient participation (Crawford et al. 2002). These concepts have attracted much attention, both in research and international and national guidelines, during the last years.

Theoretical models of care focusing on the women's perspective have been developed in different countries and maternity care settings such as in the USA (Lehrman 1988, Thompson et al. 1989, Swanson 1991, Kennedy 2000), New Zealand and Scotland (Fleming 1998, Pairman 2010), Sweden (Berg 2005, Lundgren and Berg 2007), Iceland (Halldorsdottir and Karlsdottir 2011), and South Africa (Maputle 2010). These theoretical models demonstrate similarities related to woman-centred care such as respecting human dignity and self-determination (Lehrman 1988), social support and positive presence (Thompson et al. 1989) centring the one cared for and being with (Swanson 1991), women with midwives attending (Fleming 1998), respecting and supporting the uniqueness of the woman (Kennedy 2000, Lundgren and Berg 2007), care for the unique woman (Berg 2005, Halldorsdottir and Karlsdottir 2011) and mutual participation (Maputle 2010).

Despite the similarities between the above theoretical models, differences exist related to cultural differences and professional roles. Therefore, based on previous research, a theoretical midwifery model of woman-centred care in the Nordic context (MiMo) has been developed (Berg et al. 2012). The model (Figure 5.1) has been developed based on a synthesis of 12 qualitative studies on women's and midwives' experiences of care during pregnancy and birth performed in Sweden and Iceland (Berg et al. 2012). The model includes five main themes. Three central intertwined themes are: a reciprocal relationship; a birthing atmosphere; and grounded knowledge. The remaining two themes, which likewise influence care, are: the cultural context (with hindering and promoting norms); and the balancing act involved in facilitating woman-centred care. The model has been further validated by focus group interviews in Sweden and Iceland during 2012–2013 with 30 midwives.

Grounded knowledge

Grounded knowledge involves theoretical, experienced-based and sensitive knowledge embodied in the midwife. Theoretical knowledge about various complicated conditions and diseases that may interfere with childbearing is essential as it gives midwives a feeling of security in their professional role, a presupposition for trustful guidance through the process of childbirth. What is equally essential for knowledge development is reflection by the midwife, both on her own and together with midwifery colleagues. The term 'embodied knowledge' focuses on the fact that the knowledge is integrated knowledge for the midwife. Tested and proven intuitive knowledge gives them the courage to use their intuition in relation to the individual woman at a more integrated level of embodied knowledge, promote normality and how to use elements of medical techniques. Knowledge in relation to the woman means that specific knowledge is obtained and developed by interacting with the woman herself. Consequently it is crucial for the midwife to be sensitive to every woman's needs (Berg et al. 2012). By using this knowledge the midwife can make room for spiritual questions:

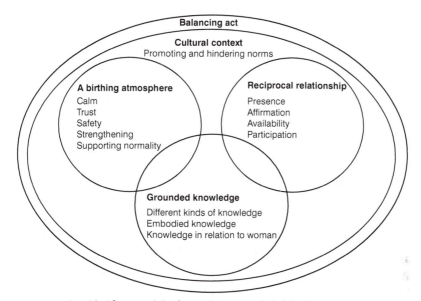

FIGURE 5.1 A midwifery model of women-centred childbirth care in Swedish and Icelandic settings (Berg, Olafsdottir, Lundgren (2012, 83))

Midwifery skills are just this … to connect with the woman … [so] that I know what I have in my hands. This is this feeling when you have become professionally skilled on some level.

(Berg et al. 2012, 85)

A birthing atmosphere

A birthing atmosphere is a place for birth that radiates calmness, trust and safety. Further, it is an atmosphere that is strengthening and that supports normality. For the woman and her partner it can give a feeling of being at home, in a mental sense 'owning' the room, feeling relaxed and 'fully there'. In a strengthening atmosphere the midwife's role is to empower the woman (Berg et al. 2012). A birthing atmosphere thereby is facilitating for the woman to express her spiritual and existential needs to the midwife (see Lemay and Hastie on birth space, Chapter 7).

Reciprocal relationship

A reciprocal relationship involves presence, affirmation, availability and participation. The midwife first needs to get to know and understand the woman – who she is and what her and her family's needs are. The first encounter is therefore of importance. Presence is the act of 'being with' the woman during childbirth. Affirmation means that the woman needs to be seen, i.e. recognised as a genuine subject. What is essential here is that the midwife feels connected to the woman and is there with and for the woman. The midwife needs to be available and it is fundamental to the midwife's learning and skill development. This includes the act of being with the woman; and of being present, open and adaptable, supporting each woman according to her unique needs. Participation for the woman means to be involved in the birth process, to have a continuous dialogue with the midwife who listens to her, informs her about the labour progress and also supports her to be responsible and make her own choices in the maternity care. For the woman, a lack of participation can create a feeling of not being in contact with the birth and of not having given birth herself (Berg et al. 2012). A reciprocal relationship involving presence, affirmation, availability and participation is a ground for encountering the individual woman's spiritual needs as she enters the journey into childbirth during the antenatal period, as this woman explains:

> I felt that they were very sensitive and I was able to be myself and could show all sides of myself and was still believed.
>
> *(Berg et al. 2012, 83)*

This reflects what Marcel (1956) says about being present with others at times of need:

> There are some people who reveal themselves as present ... when we are in pain or in need ... the person who is at my disposal is the one who is capable of being with me with the whole of himself.
>
> *(Marcel 1956, 39–40)*

Cultural context with promoting and hindering norms, and a balancing act

Finally the model consists of two overall themes: cultural context with promoting and hindering norms, and a balancing act. An accepted cultural norm is that the midwife should be at the side of the woman during labour and birth, continuously supporting her according to her needs. This is a continuous balancing act since everything can change very quickly, from being normal to being abnormal where the midwife uses her grounded knowledge. In institutional modern care a hindering norm is where a midwife is obliged to give care to more than one woman at a time. In such a situation the midwife has to go from one woman to the other giving a minimum of care and risk being mentally absent for everyone, or she can decide to be present for the one who needs it most and neglect the other (Berg et al. 2012). This is the woman's perspective in this situation:

> It felt as if she [the midwife] always came just two minutes too late ... as if half of her was still in the other room.
>
> *(Berg et al. 2012, 85)*

A balancing act means maintaining a reciprocal relationship and an optimal birthing atmosphere during the birth using grounded knowledge while handling the hindering cultural norms. This balancing is like a 'line of dancing' in a busy labour ward with simultaneous work tasks to do and time pressures; it is an environment where medico-technical philosophical values predominate and influence the rules and regulations of the labour ward. Yet the crucial thing in this balancing dance is to continually show respect for the individual woman and her unique needs.

Conclusion

In summary, pregnancy is a transition to the unknown, including meeting one's life situation, meeting something inevitable and preparing for the unknown. Further, it is a life-opening – a process of opening up different dimensions in life, and existential questions related to both suffering and power. The women may express themselves as being chosen and refer to a feeling of holiness. Pregnancy thereby influences the existence of the woman and is the starting point for a life-opening that continues during the birth. During pregnancy, healthcare professionals need to prepare women for the birth process. When entering the process of birth, encounters with others are important for the woman, both with herself and with health professionals, demanding both stillness and change. Stillness for the woman means being in the moment, exemplified as presence and being one's body. Change is expressed as transition – to the unknown and to motherhood. For the midwife, stillness and change equals being an *anchored companion*. To be a companion is to be an available person that listens to and follows the woman through the antenatal period and through the process of birth. To be anchored is to be the person who, in the birth process, respects the limits of the woman's ability as well as her own professional limits. For midwives these limits are the need to adhere to regulations and guidelines of their local maternity systems of care. For a woman it is vital that she be able to actively participate in the process and not feel limited by others. However, some women may experience a lack of participation throughout their pregnancy and birth experience and become an object for others to work upon. This chapter has shown how childbirth has the potential to strengthen self-confidence and trust in others but also be a cause of failure and distrust. Forces related to both suffering and strength may be developed, which can be explained with the concept 'border situation'. Woman-centred care involving a grounded knowledge and reciprocal relationship may facilitate focusing existential and spiritual questions during childbearing.

References

Anderson, T. 2000. Feeling safe enough to let go: The relationship between a woman and her midwife during second stage of labour. In M. Kirkham (ed.) *The midwife–woman relationship* (pp.116–143). China: Palgrave Macmillan.

Beck, C.T. 2004. Birth trauma in the eye of the beholder. *Nursing Research*, 53, 28–35.

Berg, M. 2005. A midwifery model of care for childbearing women at high risk: Genuine caring in caring for the genuine. *Journal of Perinatal Education*, 14, 9–21.

Berg, M., Lundgren, I., Hermansson, E. and Wahlberg, V. 1996. Women's experience of the encounter with the midwife during childbirth. *Midwifery*, 12, 11–15.

Berg, M., Olafsdottir, O.A. and Lundgren, I. 2012. A midwifery model of supportive care during pregnancy and childbirth in a Nordic context. *Sexual and Reproductive Healthcare*, 3, 2, 79–87.

Bergbom, I., Modh Arneklev, C., Lundgren, I. and Lindwall, L. 2016. First-time pregnant women's experiences of early pregnancy. *Scandinavian Journal of Caring Sciences*, 11 October 2016.

Bergum, V. 1997. *A child on her mind. The experience of becoming a mother.* Connecticut, CT: Bergin & Garvey.

Bondas, T. and Eriksson, K. 2001. Women's lived experiences of pregnancy: A tapestry of joy and suffering. *Qualitative Health Research,* 11, 6, 824–840.

Bryar, R. and Sinclair, M. 2011. *Theory for midwifery practice.* New York: Palgrave Macmillan.

Crawford, M. et al. 2002. Systematic review of involving patients in the planning and development of healthcare. *British Medical Journal*, 325, 1263.

Crowther, S. and Hall, J. 2015. Spirituality and spiritual care in and around childbirth. *Women and Birth*, 28, 173–178.

Davis-Floyd, R., Barclay, L. and Tritten, J. 2009. *Birth models that work.* Berkeley, CA: University of California Press.

Downe, S. 2008. *Normal childbirth: Evidence and debate.* Edinburgh: Churchill Livingstone/ Elsevier.

Ekman, I. et al. 2011. Person-centered care: Ready for prime time. *European Journal of Cardiovascular Nursing: Journal of the Working Group on Cardiovascular Nursing of the European Society of Cardiology*, 10, 4, 248–251.

Fleming, V.E. 1998. Women-with-midwives-with-women: A model of interdependence. *Midwifery*, 14, 3, 137–143.

Halldorsdottir, S. and Karlsdottir, S.I. 2011. The primacy of the good midwife in midwifery services: An evolving theory of professionalism in midwifery. *Scandinavian Journal of Caring Sciences*, 25, 4, 806–817.

Hunter, B. 2009. *Mixed messages: Midwives' experiences of managing emotion.* In B. Hunter and R. Deery (eds) *Emotions in midwifery and reproduction* (pp.175–191). NY: Palgrave Macmillan.

Jaspers, K. 1963. *Introduktion till filosofin (Introduction to philosophy).* Stockholm: Bonnier.

Kennedy, H.P. 2000. A model of exemplary midwifery practice. Results of a Delphi study. *Journal of Midwifery & Women's Health*, 45, 1, 4–19.

Lahood, G. 2007. Rumour of angels and heavenly midwives: Anthropology of transpersonal events and childbirth. *Women and Birth*, 20, 3–10.

Lehrman, E.J.A. 1988. *A theoretical framework for nurse-midwifery practice.* Tucson, AZ: University of Arizona.

Leinweber, J. and Rowe, H. J. 2010. The costs of 'being with the woman': Secondary traumatic stress in midwifery. *Midwifery*, 26, 76–87.

Lundgren, I. 2002. Releasing and relieving encounters. Experiences of pregnancy and childbirth (thesis). Uppsala University, Sweden: Faculty of medicine.

Lundgren, I. 2004. Releasing and relieving encounters – experiences of pregnancy and childbirth. *Scandinavian Journal of Caring Sciences*, 18, 368–375.

Lundgren, I. 2010a. Swedish women's experiences of doula support during childbirth. *Midwifery*, 26, 173–180.

Lundgren, I. 2010b. Experiences of wanting and searching for a home birth when professional care at home is not an option in public health care. *Sexual and Reproductive Healthcare*, 1, 61–66.

Lundgren, I. 2011. The meaning of giving birth from a long-term perspective for childbearing women. In G. Thomson, F. Dykes and S. Downe (eds) *Qualitative research in midwifery and childbirth – phenomenological approaches* (pp.115–132). London and New York: Routledge.

Lundgren, I. and Berg, M. 2007. Central concepts in the midwife–woman relationship. *Scandinavian Journal of Caring Sciences*, 21, 220–228.

Lundgren, I. and Dahlberg, K. 1998. Women's experience of pain during childbirth. *Midwifery*, 14, 105–110.

Lundgren, I. and Dahlberg, K. 2002. Midwives' experience of the encounter with women and their pain during childbirth. *Midwifery*, 2, 155–164.

Lundgren, I. and Wahlberg, V. 1999. The experience of pregnancy: A hermeneutical/phenomenological study. *The Journal of Perinatal Education*, 3, 12–20.

Lundgren, I., Karlsdottir, I. and Bondas, T. 2009. Long-term memories and experiences of childbirth in a Nordic context – a secondary analysis. *International Journal of Qualitative Studies on Health and Well-being*, 4, 115–128.

Maputle, M.S. 2010. A woman-centred childbirth model. *Health SA Gesondheid*, 15, 1, 8.

Marcel, G. 1956. *The philosophy of existentialism*. New York: Citadel Press.

Maslow, A. 1979. *Religion, values and peak experiences*. New York: Viking.

Modh, C., Lundgren, I. and Bergbom, I. 2011. First time pregnant women's experiences in early pregnancy. *Journal of Qualitative Studies on Health and Well-being*, 6, 5600.

Nilsson, C., Bondas, T. and Lundgren, I. 2010. Previous birth experience in women with intense fear of childbirth. *Journal of Obstetric, Gynecologic & Neonatal Nursing*, 39, 3, 298–309.

Nilsson, C., Lundgren, I., Karlström, A. and Hildingsson, I. 2012. Self-reported fear of childbirth and its association with women´s birth experience and mode of delivery: A longitudinal population-based study. *Women and Birth*, 25, 114–121.

Olsson, P. 2000. *Antenatal midwifery consultations*. (thesis) Department of Nursing, Umeå University, Sweden.

Pairman, S. 2010. *Midwifery partnership: A professionalizing strategy for midwives*. In M. Kirkham (ed.) *The midwife–mother relationship* (pp.208–231). Basingstoke: Palgrave Macmillan.

Pembroke, N. and Pembroke, J. 2008. The spirituality of presence in midwifery care, *Midwifery*, 24, 321–327.

Rooks, J. P. 1999. The midwifery model of care. *Journal of Nurse-Midwifery*, 44, 370–374.

Sandall, J., Soltani, H., Gates, S. and Shennan, A., 2016. *Midwife-led continuity models versus other models of care for childbearing women*. Cochrane Database of Systematic Reviews 28, 4:CD004667.

Swanson, K.M. 1991. Empirical development of a middle range theory of caring. *Nursing Research*, 40, 3, 161–166.

Thompson, J.E., Oakley, D., Burke, M., Jay, S. and Conklin, M. 1989. Theory building in nurse midwifery. The care process. *Journal of Nurse-Midwifery*, 34, 3, 120–130.

6

PREGNANCY LOSS AND COMPLEXITY

Joan Gabrielle Lalor

Although the literature is replete with references to birth as sacred, a spiritual journey where a new life is welcomed into the world, this is juxtaposed with the almost exclusively medical focus on birth if something should go wrong. Ultrasound screening for foetal anomalies was first introduced into practice more than thirty years ago, and rapid technological developments have meant that women's experience of pregnancy has changed irrevocably. While science endeavours to come to terms with constantly evolving diagnostic techniques, mass screening of foetal health in pregnancy is blurring the traditional boundaries between health and illness, as normal populations are being screened for a condition that has not manifested itself through the identification of risk factors. Acceptance of routine ultrasound in low risk pregnancy has led to the modality developing a social meaning, one that for many women has come to dominate its medical use (Lalor 2007). Attending to a routine second trimester ultrasound examination is perceived as an opportunity to meet the baby, as visualisation of the foetus not only enhances parental attachment; the recorded images also facilitate a sharing of the experience with friends and families (Lalor 2007).

There is little doubt that one of the most profound inequities for parents eagerly awaiting the birth of their child is to have their hopes and dreams shattered by the diagnosis of a severe or lethal abnormality. The evidence is unequivocal in that women have demonstrated that a threat to foetal health represents a major traumatic event (Lalor, Devane and Begley 2007) – one in which their assumptions and beliefs about the world are violated. So why is an adverse diagnosis so traumatic?

I have spent many years as a clinician imparting a diagnosis to couples, followed by many more listening to their stories as a researcher. My work in this field has been exclusively within the Republic of Ireland, a country with a complicated history of religious involvement in State affairs, where the influence of Church doctrine on social policy is well documented (Inglis 1998). Smyth (2005) suggests that our political and national identity is constructed in traditional, patriarchal, familial and orthodoxly catholic terms. In Ireland, Church and State have been intertwined for many decades and the integration of catholic philosophy and state policy is well documented (Oaks 1999, 2003). Catholic doctrine is interwoven into the Constitution that sets out how Ireland is to be governed (Government of Ireland 1999). For example, Article 40.3.3 offers constitutional protection to the unborn, stating that the unborn has an equal right to life to the mother, clearly indicating that Ireland has a national identity that is unambiguously pro-life. Consequently, women who are pregnant in Ireland are aware that termination of pregnancy remains out of the State remit, leaving women with a feeling that choosing not to continue the pregnancy is inherently wrong (Lalor 2013). Therefore it is unsurprising to find many women continue the pregnancy in order to have family support or because they simply do not have the wherewithal to access services outside of the State (Lalor 2007). For those that choose to travel, they do so in a context of secrecy and lies (Lalor 2013). In this chapter I will use women's stories that participated in my doctoral and postdoctoral work to illustrate the psychological burden associated with a diagnosis of foetal anomaly in pregnancy and how a belief in God (or other higher power) influenced their ability to cope.

I have found the theoretical construct of the Assumptive World conceived by Colin Murray Parkes to be indispensable in my efforts to understand the psychosocial process experienced by those affected. Colin Murray Parkes (1971) defines the assumptive world in terms of

the only world we know and it includes everything we know or think we know. It includes our interpretation of the past and our own expectation of the future, our plans and our prejudices. Any or all of these may need to change as a result of changes in the life space.

(Parkes 1971, 102)

Without exception, receiving an adverse prenatal diagnosis constitutes a change in one's expectations and plans for a pregnancy. Seldom are accounts available from those affected by prenatal diagnosis. In this chapter I explore whether spirituality and faith are evident in the narratives of those who hope to adapt to an unforeseen and at times unpredictable future, as previously unquestioned beliefs of normality are replaced with shattered assumptions (Parkes 1971).

Although women universally accept routine ultrasound in pregnancy, understanding the meaning of an adverse diagnosis requires some exploration of the context. In many countries where routine ultrasound is available, there is a high incidence of spiritual and religious beliefs in the population being screened. In the 2011 Census in Ireland, although a surge in the number of people that describe themselves as non-religious was evident at 5.6%, just over 84% described themselves as Catholic, and the remaining 10% as affiliated to other religious groupings. Although figures vary internationally, there remain higher proportions of the population who indicate religious association, as over 76% of citizens in North America and 59.3% in the United Kingdom are affiliated to Christian faiths, with many others describing themselves as non-religious. In considering these census figures, it is important not to confuse spirituality and religion as not everyone who considers himself or herself religious consider themselves spiritual and vice versa (see Chapter 1). The supposition that society is fast becoming a secular one is highly contested, as there seems to be little correlation between attendance at church and belief in God. Consequently, statistical patterns indicating a decline in membership or attendance in traditional religious practices does not necessarily indicate a non-belief in the existence of God or a higher power. Therefore it is important to consider the distinction between religion and spirituality as many who describe themselves as non-religious may engage in spiritual coping activities such as prayer or pleading with God in time of stress.

For the purpose of this chapter, spirituality will be conceived as an attempt to seek meaning and purpose in life in relation to a higher power, a universal force or God. The word spirituality is derived from the Latin word *spirale*, to blow or to breathe, thus denoting giving breath or hope to individuals, families or communities. Religion on the other hand refers to a form of social institution, an agreed set of beliefs with accompanying practices and rituals, and can play a significant role in helping individuals to cope with stressful life events (Janoff-Bulman 1992).

The positions outlined below have evolved over the course of my professional career, in the capacities of clinician, academic and researcher, as I have had occasion to work with many couples traumatised by an unexpected diagnosis of a serious or lethal foetal anomaly in pregnancy. In my doctoral and postdoctoral work I used a grounded theory approach to explore women's experiences of an adverse prenatal diagnosis. Over sixty women were interviewed on up to three occasions from the diagnosis up to and beyond the birth. Narratives from these interviews will be used as exemplars of how women whose lives are disrupted by a profound loss seek to make sense of this ostensibly meaningless event.

Diagnosis of foetal anomaly – a violation of the assumptive world

Regularising second trimester ultrasound has created an environment where women attend to seek reassurance of presumed foetal well-being rather than the exclusion or confirmation of foetal abnormality. Although most infants are born well, approximately 1:50 will be born with a structural abnormality and 1:700 with a chromosomal or serious genetic disorder. As the presence of a foetal anomaly is relatively uncommon, women are not prepared for such a diagnosis, in particular when the pregnancy has been without complication up to that point. Consequently, when the expectation of normality was devastated through an adverse diagnosis, some mothers were not only incredulous but also questioned how they could have been visited by such an injustice. Several systematic reviews have found that the use of religious and spiritual coping efforts are associated with better emotional outcomes (Frankl 1963). In my doctoral and postdoctoral work I sought to explore not just the initial response to the diagnosis but how women made decisions regarding the outcome of the pregnancy, and in particular, how they adapted to this traumatic and unexpected news. All of the narrative quotes are excerpts from interviews I undertook with women during the course of my work (Lalor, Begley and Galavan 2009, Lalor 2013, Lalor, Devane and Begley 2007, Lalor and Begley 2005, 2006). For some women the initial response to the news may be disbelief, as some resorted to prayer (Janoff-Bulman 1992), hoping that it is all a terrible mistake. Sian said:

> I mean it happens to people [conceiving a baby with an abnormality], like you think it will never happen, but like I mean these things do happen and then you have to think about them. If I was to think about why it would seriously drag me down through the pregnancy if I was to, sort of get hung up on it like. ... I lost my child for about four days [after the diagnosis] and it was like a big black cloud and you wake up in the morning and you think I can't get out of this ... So I thank God, I just hand it over to the Lord, like and say well, you know, God give me the grace or the strength, or please God the baby will be perfect.
>
> *(Lalor 2007, 129)*

Sian's ultrasound had indicated the possibility of duodenal atresia and Sian was given a 1:3 risk that her baby had Down syndrome. Although it has been shown that spiritual beliefs can interfere with medical help seeking behaviours, in the context of prenatal diagnosis this behaviour manifested most often in a refusal to undergo invasive testing, such as amniocentesis. Refusing further testing was seen as a way to keep the hope of a healthy baby alive. Sian refused amniocentesis as she needed to keep the hope that the baby did not have Down syndrome in order to cope on a day-to-day basis until the birth.

> I said no, it [the amniocentesis result] could put a totally different outlook on the last few months of your pregnancy; we prefer to think that the baby will be normal ... I feel what we have to focus on is getting our head around it, keep going with the ordinary everyday things. We hope to cope, hope that the baby will feed and sleep ... that we will become normal.
>
> *(Lalor 2007, 186)*

In the field of positive psychology it has been recognised that negative orientations toward the future are associated with hopelessness and pessimism. Therefore in order to maintain hope, positive expectations and the cognitive capacity to direct one's thoughts towards a future goal (in Sian's case a healthy baby) is central to an individual's ability to manage successfully that which was unforeseen. Although Sian had a strong belief in God and engaged in spiritually based activities such as attending Mass and praying for strength and support, others used their faith as a way of coming to terms with the fact that they might never find a reason for why this has happened. Emma said:

> You know, I am not a religious person but I do talk to God and that … and I do say well you wouldn't want me to go through this would you? Maybe He [God] wants me to go through this. Just telling yourself, maybe this is to be, and just get on with it.
>
> *(Lalor 2007, 151)*

Some even viewed the diagnosis as a wake-up call to live a better life (Becker et al. 2007, Gall et al. 2005), such as taking this event as a signal to eat more healthily, avoid risk-taking behaviours, reduce alcohol intake or to stop smoking. I was prompted to search further as to why some women believed that this unforeseen event could be attributable to their own actions. It was a quote from Emma about the unfairness of the diagnosis that led me to Lerner's theory of 'belief in a just world' (Lerner 1980). Lerner's (1980) just-world hypothesis is based on the assumption that a person's actions are inherently inclined to bring just and fitting consequences. Evidence of this belief in the vernacular in Ireland (and likely elsewhere) include common parlance such as 'you reap what you sow', 'what goes around comes around' and 'your chickens have come home to roost'.

Therefore in the case of very negative events, people may often find it easier to attribute blame rather than accept the randomness or unjustness of the experience. Although uncommon, some women chose to blame themselves. Fiona had two healthy children and had just received a diagnosis of hydrocephaly in her third pregnancy.

> I would blame a lot of it on the wine. There is a difference between liking wine and loving wine, I love wine … I would drink a bottle no problem. I wouldn't have a problem with it in the world. But like you see on my first pregnancy I couldn't drink. But then when I had [second baby], I didn't drink on that pregnancy, I drank beer or whatever but I went to wine then, you know [in this pregnancy]. But I blame it on me, and then I try to blame it on like loads of things, but mainly me.
>
> *(Lalor 2007, 148)*

Hayley, a single mother with a two year old son described how she discovered she was pregnant following her return from a holiday with her family.

> I blamed myself. I was in New York with my best friend and my Mam and my aunt and I was out on the batter every night. I was getting drunk. I was a week over there and I found out I was pregnant.
>
> *(Lalor 2007, 149)*

One aspect of constructing meaning is to seek significance in the event, to re-prioritise, and to learn lessons for the future. Both Fiona and Hayley attributed the diagnosis to their alcohol intake in early pregnancy. Each indicated that in attributing causality to their behaviour they could protect themselves in future pregnancies by doing things differently. Lerner (cited in Miller and Kelley 2005) suggests that in order to maintain an illusion of control over a random event it is tempting to attribute blame as this keeps the 'belief in a just world' intact, restoring one's sense of control, and avoiding the significant cognitive task of revising one's assumptions about the world. However, some women, who did not blame themselves for the diagnosis, felt, on occasion, that their friends were attributing them with causal responsibility for the anomaly through actions that they may have taken or failed to take earlier in the pregnancy. Ava, whose baby was diagnosed with a lethal abdominal wall defect, commented on how friends were keen to get to the root of the problem:

> That was Christmas day, a friend of mine called, I mean she is genuine no more than anybody else has been about the whole thing and she was saying to me, so they just don't know why it's happening? I mean we have asked this question ourselves and they [foetal medicine specialists] just don't know why it would happen, and it's just sporadic. So I just said nothing to her, I just let it go. But she turned around and said to me I know it makes no difference but did you check if you were pregnant say when we went to [a friend's party] and you had a couple of glasses of wine and maybe you didn't know you were pregnant? I am looking at her thinking I know it has nothing to do with that but even suggesting that there is any element of blame … we haven't spoken since.
>
> *(Lalor 2007, 149)*

Lerner (1980) suggests that just as we believe in a just world so do others around us. Therefore if Ava was not to blame for the diagnosis this may have threatened her friend's security around conceiving a normal baby. However, for others the sense of injustice and distress caused them to turn away from their religious beliefs and forsake their beliefs, temporarily if not permanently.

Keeping the faith in an unjust world – it's more than a spiritual struggle

Rotter (1966) proposed that individuals have an internal locus of control – a belief that what happens to us is a consequence of our actions. However, when the trauma experienced does not fit with this assumption, the individual becomes an 'innocent victim' and may become overwhelmed by the objectively uncontrollable nature of the crisis. Molly prepared assiduously for her first pregnancy, refraining from taking alcohol, altering her diet and taking pre-conceptual folic acid, yet Molly received a diagnosis of anencephaly.

So I don't know, part of me thinks like I did everything so right and yet it went so wrong. It's weird. Maybe if … there is something about doing everything so correct, you know, I know it would have anyway but it is a thought that goes through my mind like when you are so adamantly balancing your food and things and it still happened. The same for folic acid I am just almost, I feel so let down, you are let down by everything, you are let down by God, you're let down by your body.

(Lalor 2007, 186)

Other elements of the assumptive world such as 'I am a good person, things are meant to be a certain way, God is good, having a vision of the future' also emerged during women's reconstruction of their experience. This is similar to the premise outlined in Lerner's (1980) theory of 'belief in a just world' such as 'bad things happen to bad people'.

Emma's diagnosis in the context of having prepared for pregnancy violated her belief that she could have some control over future outcomes.

They [the staff] said just go out and get a bit of a breather, I got a bit angry then, you know. I know it's terrible, I am not a bad person but I was coming down the steps in the main building, coming down the steps and going out and watching all the girls either going off with their babies, husbands coming in, partners coming in with the carry cot to bring the baby home, and there was one girl parked outside. I always looked towards that day when I would be bringing my baby home … and young girls were going in for their appointments … Here they are going in no problem, getting everything handed to them, perfect babies probably. Because I had felt I had done everything by the book. You know, I don't smoke and very rarely drink, look after myself as much as I can, you know, as you do, well I always do try and eat well and whatever. I think I tried to do everything right in life, you know, not do anything wrong on anybody or you know, and was thinking this is unfair like for us … it should be them.

(Lalor 2007, 132)

Emma's experience shakes her beliefs and provides her with evidence that supports the fact that the world may not be just. Making sense of loss requires a search for meaning, and one of the first steps in this journey was for women to seek answers to the 'Why me?' question through gaining information to clarify and assess the consequences of the diagnosis for the pregnancy/baby. Meaning is an explanation for an event that renders it consistent with one's assumptions or understanding of the nature of the social world. That is, an event 'makes sense' or 'has meaning' when it does not contradict fundamental beliefs about justice, order and the distribution of outcomes (Rotter 1966). Some of the most common questions asked as women seek meaning in the immediate aftershock of the diagnosis are: Why did this happen? Why me? Will it be ok? What caused this?

When solace in prayers or an acceptance of God's will does not give sufficient explanation to the event, some experienced a type of spiritual struggle, in particular, if God was viewed as punitive or failing to respond to pleas for help. Lori was pregnant with her second baby and was a mother to a healthy two year old daughter. The ultrasound detected a serious cardiac defect and Lori, unlike Sian, accepted the offer of amniocentesis to confirm or exclude a diagnosis of Down syndrome, as she described not knowing as 'torture'.

> The day mm … I got the results she has Downs there is this big church there beside [hospital] and I went in and I walked back out. This is not for me; I know my faith is gone now.
>
> *(Lalor 2007, 151)*

When asked if Lori practised her faith before the diagnosis she replied:

> Yes, I was brought up Catholic and maybe I prayed at night. I haven't been to Mass for a while though. Oh I was very angry, very, very angry. I mean I am sure I was saying what did I do to deserve this? I have no faith now. I had to sit in Mass one day, I wanted to go for my granny's anniversary but just listening to the priest standing up there, you know the way they talk and lecture us, and I was so angry. My baby might die and the way I am looking at it is and here is my faith coming again that if she died God is after taking her away … why take her back?
>
> *(Lalor 2007, 151)*

Irrespective of whether women mentioned a belief in God or not, they all said that they had to have hope (in something) to cope. This may have been simply that when the baby had a lethal anomaly they hoped that the baby could be born alive in order to be baptised. Laoise said:

> I hope that he is born alive and really hope for as long as possible he will live. The longer time I can get with him the better, but I need to bond now, while he is alive, just in case [he is stillborn]. It's hard to let go. I mean just, like I really want to bond with him and have him for as long as possible.
>
> *(Lalor 2007, 152)*

Heather, whose baby had been diagnosed with a lethal cloacal abnormality, said:

> I have asked for a section so she can be born alive; she can't be baptised if she is stillborn.
>
> *(Lalor 2007, 124)*

For others, the prospect of caring for a child with significant challenges was the worst possible outcome, and in these cases women often prayed for the best possible outcome, and for some death before birth was the preferred ending. Niamh said:

> I have heard it over and over again, yes I know I shouldn't be wanting it to be over and I really do still want to think the best for the baby but dear God I am thinking how in God's name am I going to get through the next few weeks, I am hoping things won't be half as bad as what I expect. But from the day you get pregnant you hope your baby will be fine now I hope it will be the least bad problem.
>
> *(Lalor 2007, 180)*

Doireann, on the other hand, was fearful that she might not be able to cope with caring for a child with complex needs:

> I'm hoping they'll say the heartbeat is fading away. My biggest fear is that the baby will survive and I'll be left with a seriously handicapped baby ... How will I cope?
>
> *(Lalor 2007, 110)*

When women described themselves in negative self-deprecating terms such as 'I deserve this or this is my punishment' feelings akin to unworthiness or worthlessness emerged.

> I am sick of hearing God sent you this child ... then I met a lovely priest yesterday just out of blue walking down the street, like I felt dirty and I suddenly felt this is my punishment and like he doesn't know me or what is going on (that my baby is abnormal and I don't want him) ... I am not even Catholic and I still feel dirty.
>
> *(Lalor 2007, 176)*

Regan understood that termination of pregnancy was not available in Ireland and was clearly viewed as immoral; however, as she had been sharing care with her GP she chose to inform her out of courtesy of her decision to travel.

> I found her incredibly good till I told her I had a baby with anencephaly and I was planning on going to England ... and I just didn't like her reaction ... You see I understand as well that they can't give any information, they can't give their opinion, they can't but ... But she could be humane I sort of feel that she thought I should have gone to term ... she told me how dare I say such a thing and asked me to leave.
>
> *(Lalor 2007, 172)*

Although women are aware of the legal context, they assume medical professionals will put their personal beliefs aside in the context of a consultation.

To be faced with such opprobrium by a health professional adds to the guilt and shame women are made to feel that they would even consider such a heinous act. For those that continued the pregnancy, some women were so overwhelmed by the news and an inability to see a future in which they could cope, that they used avoidant coping strategies, sometimes not leaving the house for days. Cliona said:

> I was still tossing at maybe three this morning, I still hadn't closed me eyes, and I know he [her partner] only went to sleep at about one, but we weren't, we weren't talking about it. When he went to sleep last night I probably cried for a little while all right … I haven't been out in days … I just don't want to see anyone.
>
> *(Lalor 2007, 128)*

Irrespective of whether women at an individual level describe themselves as religious or not, when faced with the prospect of caring for a baby with significant health needs, or a stillbirth or neonatal death, many consider if they have the strength to cope with continuing the pregnancy. It has been previously identified that religiosity is also significant in women's decision making in terms of whether to continue the pregnancy or not (Lerner 1980). However, given the high levels of religious affiliation and spirituality in the Irish population, these women were asked if their decision to continue or to terminate the pregnancy was influenced by a particular belief system. Laura said:

> Surprisingly not, I thought it might, you know … but it hasn't for me. I don't feel, I don't feel I am sending the baby to hell or anything (by having a termination); I am not worried about that. I am more worried about it suffering, its physical suffering than its soul suffering. I am not sure if it has a soul, I really am not. I am not sure how conscious it is of what is happening to it and it's hard to imagine that, and the God I believe in is not that kind of God [who would punish her for this decision], He is not so merciless I think.
>
> *(Lalor 2007, 173)*

Finding meaning in the aftermath of an adverse prenatal diagnosis

References to God and the belief in a just world were common in women's narratives. Some described trying to come to terms with the diagnosis as a spiritual struggle as they questioned why God was punishing them when they perceived that they were not responsible for the diagnosis. For others, prayer was used as a form of bargaining to seek a better outcome or as a way to find strength to carry their burden. Although women made reference to more frequent conversations with God, none reported an increased involvement with the church, as they did not perceive that this would help them to cope. An overwhelming belief that God could remedy the situation was rare, and references to one's faith being shaken or lost were common. Surprisingly, although references to a belief in their God were common in everyday language, only one woman had a faith so strong that she believed that a miracle was possible if she prayed hard enough.

Neimeyer et al. (2002) contend that human beings are 'meaning makers' as we seek to interpret our experiences in order to find a purpose and significance in the event. Following a traumatic event such as the diagnosis of a serious or lethal foetal abnormality, basic assumptions about the world, such as, *parents do not outlive their children* and *bad things happen to bad people* are shattered. For many, the search for meaning that follows seeks to resolve and restore previously held assumptions. For some, attributions of blame are used as a mechanism to restore our previously held assumptions, by altering our behaviour, we can alter the outcome and regain control of the future. The literature offers many examples of how individuals in the wake of a traumatic event have used their religious beliefs, faith and spiritual activities as a means of finding meaning and coping.

Although my research did not seek to measure if women of religion coped better with the loss than non-religious women, the findings show that the more demanding searches for meaning are associated with prolonged feelings of injustice, unfairness and loss of control. In this context it is more likely that women will experience a sense of helplessness and hopelessness with little attention focused on the future. Without hope, the pain of the loss can become overwhelming, resulting in self-isolation and potentially despair. Just as some women accommodated the diagnosis easily into their assumptive worlds, some may never find meaning, but other adjustment variables such as somatic effects, negativity levels and future mindedness can be monitored by caregivers and appropriate referrals made if concerns develop, as complicated grief is not a self-limiting process (Zisook and DeVaul 1983). A more recent finding, supported by a growing evidence base, is that complicated grief reactions go together with a sense of pervasive hopelessness.

The term hope has a long history, and according to the pagan Greek myth, hope was the only good force to be contained in Pandora's Box. In the past, the Biblical St Paul exalted Hope as one of the most fundamental Christian virtues, while Dante equated the absence of hope with hell (Stroebe, van Son and Stroebe 2000). In principle, hope has been referred to as a positive expectation, a wish about an issue which has a realistic prospect of coming to pass (Magaletta and Oliver 1999). However a darker side to hope such as blind hope, false hope (Peterson and Seligman 2004) and so on, may exist.[1] Consequently, hope has been presented in binary terms within philosophical debate as both 'a blessing and a curse' (Snyder et al. 2002). In the context of foetal anomaly diagnosis, as the assumption of foetal health is lost, one strategy utilised by women to reconstruct their assumptive world was to hope for the best possible outcome. For those women who continued the pregnancy, some hoped the outcome would be better than predicted, for others they hoped the foetus would die in utero, and for some wishing to have their baby baptised, the hope the baby would be born alive. For those who travelled outside the State to access termination of pregnancy services, women spoke of how they desperately hoped that one day they could be open about their decision and their sentiments are reflected in Laura's comment 'I wanted everyone to know something awful had happened to me – not that I did something awful'.

Finding a responsive other

Of importance to caregivers is the relationship between hope and help. There is evidence in the literature that a person can sustain his or her own hope to a certain degree; however, this cannot continue *ad infinitum* (Snyder, Cheavens and Michael 1999, 205), as hope seeks for and depends upon external sources for sustenance (Cutcliffe 2004). Within the area of palliative care it has been suggested that nurses have a crucial role as an external source in promoting hope in their patients (DuFault and Martocchio 1985), as hope is seamlessly interlaced with caring (Cutcliffe 1996). When any hope for neonatal survival was untenable, women shifted their goal and welcomed the opportunity to plan a funeral service, to do something practical for their child. Offering pathways to become involved in such endeavours was particularly useful, as it maintained a vision of the future, one where parents could have some influence.

An important change in grief theory development is the recognition of the importance of continuing bonds with the one who is lost. The notion of 'letting go' is being re-evaluated as maintaining a symbolic link with the deceased can be of more help than a hindrance. Many women spoke of loving the baby they dreamed of, the life they thought their baby would have, and so having a place or symbols of remembrance are important in the grief process. Therefore funerals and remembrance ceremonies can play a significant role. One key benefit of engagement in spiritual coping activities is that adaptive coping is mediated through a greater use of social support such as being heard, feeling loved and valued by others (Cutcliffe 1996, 1995, Cutcliffe and Grant 2001), thus caregivers play a key role at this vulnerable time.

The scope for a dedicated support role to be influential in instilling a higher sense of control in women is boundless. In addition to fostering a sense of benevolence, meaningfulness and self-worth, reassuring women that others have experienced an increase in negative thoughts, and that these thoughts are not only realistic but are extremely common (Janoff-Bulman 1992), reduces the sense of isolation that women experience. However, perhaps the strength of a dedicated support role lies in increasing women's sense of control through accessibility; if women know they have a contact person, someone on their side to speak to, non-judgemental, who can be truly present as they construct their post-trauma narrative. Reciprocity inspires hope, and a significant negative life event such as prenatal diagnosis requires cognitive and emotional re-adjustment as women's desire to contribute to the world by nurturing a capable and caring child are threatened or crushed (Robinson and Fleming 1992), challenging our sense of who we are (Archer 1999).

Planning a pregnancy in the future was a clear indicator that women were making positive progress in rebuilding their assumptive world. Their capacity to revise their beliefs about the world predicated on what the diagnosis meant for them as individuals, and as members of a family and society. Although women are forever changed by this event, many have said they emerge 'sadder but wiser' but determined to hope for a better future. Kerrie frames it beautifully in the following quote:

> We have been to hell and back you know. We may never get pregnant again, but if we do I know I have 16–17 weeks of hell … it takes the magic out of it … but you know they say if it doesn't kill you it makes you stronger, so it just makes us appreciate how lucky we are.
>
> *(Lalor 2007, 189)*

The interconnections between traumatic loss and meaning making are undeniable, and an adverse prenatal diagnosis is a profound event that disrupts the life course of those affected. However, the relationship between religions and spiritual beliefs and the ability to find meaning in an effort to cope in the aftermath of a prenatal diagnosis requires further investigation.

Note

1 Although some women spoke in terms of hoping for a miracle, that the diagnosis would be erroneous or that the baby would die, none were deluded into believing that the particular outcome was possible. Rather it appeared to be a strategy to help the individual to get through the day.

References

Archer, J. 1999. *The Nature of Grief: The Evolution and Psychology of Reactions to Loss.* New York: Routledge.

Becker, G., Xander, C.J., Blum, H.E., Lutterbach, J., Momm, F., Gysels, M. and Higginson, I.J. 2007. 'Do religious or spiritual beliefs influence bereavement? A systematic review.' *Palliative Medicine* 21:201–217.

Cutcliffe, J.R. 1995. 'How do nurses inspire and instil hope in terminally ill HIV patients?' *Journal of Advanced Nursing* 22 (5):888–895.

Cutcliffe, J.R. 1996. 'Critically ill patients' perspectives of hope.' *British Journal of Nursing* 5 (11):687–690.

Cutcliffe, J.R. 2004. 'The inspiration of hope in bereavement counseling.' *Issues in Mental Health Nursing* 25 (2):165–190.

Cutcliffe, J.R. and Grant, G. 2001. 'What are the principles and processes of inspiring hope in cognitively impaired older adults within a continuing care environment?' *Journal of Psychiatric and Mental Health Nursing* 8 (5):427–436.

DuFault, K. and Martocchio, B.C. 1985. 'Hope – its spheres and dimensions.' *Nursing Clinics of North America* 20 (2):379–391.

Frankl, V. 1963. *Man's Search for Meaning.* Revised edn. New York: Pocket Press.

Gall, T.L., Charbonneau, C., Clarke, N.H., Grant, K., Joseph, A. and Shouldice, C. 2005. 'Understanding the nature and role of spirituality in relation to coping and health: A conceptual framework.' *Canadian Psychology* 46:88–104.

Government of Ireland. 1999. *Constitution of Ireland 1937.* Dublin: Government Publications Office.

Inglis, T. 1998. *Moral Monopoly: The Rise and Fall of the Catholic Church in Modern Ireland.* 2nd edn. Dublin: University College Dublin Press.

Janoff-Bulman, R. 1992. *Shattered Assumptions: Towards a New Psychology of Trauma.* New York: The Free Press.

Lalor, J.G. 2007. 'Recasting Hope: A Longitudinal study of women's experiences of carrying a baby with a foetal abnormality up to the birth and beyond.' PhD, School of Nursing and Midwifery University of Dublin, Trinity College.

Lalor, J. 2013. 'Thirty years after Article 40.3.3: Ireland is to legislate finally for termination of pregnancy.' *MIDIRS Midwifery Digest* 23 (2):187–192.

Lalor, J. and Begley, C. 2005. Reconstructing the future: Women's adjustment to the diagnosis of foetal abnormality. In *27th Congress of the International Confederation of Midwives.* Brisbane, Australia: ICM.

Lalor, J. and Begley, C. 2006. 'Foetal anomaly screening: what do women *want* to know?' *Journal of Advanced Nursing* 55 (1):11–19.

Lalor, J., Devane, D. and Begley, C. 2007. 'Unexpected diagnosis of foetal abnormality: Women's encounters with caregivers.' *Birth* 34 (1):80–88.

Lalor, J., Begley, C. and Galavan, E. 2009. 'Recasting Hope: a process of adaptation following fetal anomaly diagnosis.' *Social Science and Medicine* 68 (3):462–72.

Lerner, M.J. 1980. *The Belief in a Just World.* New York: Plenum.

Magaletta, P.R. and Oliver, J.M. 1999. 'The hope construct, will and ways: Their relations with self-efficacy, optimism, and general well-being.' *Journal of Clinical Psychology* 55 (5):539–551.

McIntosh, D.N., Silver, R.C. and Wortman, C.B. 1993. 'Religion's role in adjustment to a negative life event: Coping with the loss of a child.' *Journal of Personality and Social Psychology* 65:812–821.

Michenbaum, D. 2006. 'Resilience and post-traumatic growth: A constructive narrative perspective.' In *Handbook of Post-Traumatic Growth: Research and Practice,* edited by L.G. Calhaun and R.G. Tedeschi. Washington, DC: American Psychological Association.

Miller, C. and Kelley, B. 2005. 'Relationships of religiosity and spirituality with mental health and psychopathology.' In *Handbook of the psychology of religion and spirituality,* edited by R. Paloutzian and C. Parks, pp. 460–478. New York: Guildford Press.

Neimeyer, R.A., Botella, L., Herrero, O., Pacheco, M., Figureas, S. and Werner-Wildner, L.A. 2002. 'The meaning of your absence.' In *Loss of The Assumptive World. A Theory of Traumatic Loss,* edited by J. Kauffman, 31–48. New York: Brunner-Routledge.

Oaks, L. 1999. 'Irish trans/national politics and locating foetales.' In *Foetal Subjects, Feminist Positions,* edited by L.M. Morgan and M.W. Michaels, 175–198. Philadelphia, PA: Pennsylvania University Press.

Oaks, L. 2003. 'Antiabortion positions and young women's life plans in contemporary Ireland.' *Social Science & Medicine* 56 (2):1973–1986.

Parkes, C.M. 1971. 'Psycho-social transition: A field of study.' *Social Science and Medicine* 5:101–115.

Parkes, C.M. 1988. 'Bereavement as a psychosocial transition: Processes of adaptation to change.' *Journal of Social Issues* 44 (3):53–65.

Peterson, C. and Seligman, M.E.P. 2004. 'Hope (optimism, future-mindedness, future orientation).' In *Character, Strengths and Virtues. A Handbook and Classification*, edited by C. Peterson and M.E.P. Seligman, 569–624. Oxford: Oxford University Press.

Robinson, P.J. and Fleming, S. 1992. 'Depressotypic cognitive patterns in major depression and conjugal bereavement.' *Omega* 25 (4):291–305.

Rotter, J. 1966. 'Generalized expectancies for internal vs. external control of reinforcement.' *Psychological Monographs* 80 (1):(Whole No 609).

Smyth, L. 2005. *Abortion and Nation. The Politics of Reproduction in Contemporary Ireland.* Aldershot: Ashgate.

Snyder, C.R., Cheavens, J. and Michael, S.T. 1999. 'Hoping.' In *Coping*, edited by C.R. Snyder, 205–227. Oxford: Oxford University Press.

Snyder, C.R., Rand, K.L., King, E.A., Feldman, D.B. and Woodward, J.T. 2002. '"False" Hope.' *Journal of Clinical psychology* 58 (9):1003–1022.

Stroebe, M.S., van Son, M. and Stroebe, W. 2000. 'On the classification and diagnosis of pathological grief.' *Clinical Psychology Review* 20 (1):57–75.

Zisook, S. and DeVaul, R.A. 1983. 'Grief, unresolved grief and depression.' *Psychosomatics* 24 (3):247–256.

7

HOLDING SACRED SPACE IN LABOUR AND BIRTH

Céline Lemay and Carolyn Hastie

Preamble

This chapter is the offspring of two midwives from different ends of the earth, Céline from French-speaking Canada and Carolyn from Australia. Although Céline's mother tongue is French she also speaks and writes well in English while Carolyn's first language is English with only snippets of the French language. Before the actual writing began, we met weekly for several months using Skype. Our conversations ranged from the practical matters of co-writing, through various philosophical ideas, our research interests and conundrums to spirituality related topics. We shared stories about our experiences in midwifery practice. We used our stories, as midwives always do, to illustrate points in our discussion. The goal of these meetings was to learn from each other and come to a shared understanding of terms and definitions. The results of those discussions are to be found in the table of definitions (see Table 7.1); our individual voices are named in the text. While much of the content is referenced, some of the information and understandings we share in this chapter come from our vast experience in one-to-one midwifery care and reflect our learning from the women and families we were privileged to midwife and the academic work we have done in this area. The stories in this chapter come from our practice. Names of women, their locations and some elements of the stories have been changed to maintain confidentiality and anonymity for the women and their families.

Introduction

Every second, more than four babies are born on our planet. It could give the impression that birth is an ordinary event if it happens that often. But anyone who has given birth or was present at a birth will say the contrary: birth is *not* an 'ordinary' event. Birth is the beginning of any human existence and the fundamental event creating families, tribes, communities, nations. It is special, unique as well as universal. Consequently, in every place of birth and every circumstance there is a space, a sacred space for this event, where human beings are meeting their personal and shared mystery that reveals itself through many tensions: strength and fragility, love and fear, head and heart, sacred and profane, instant and eternity, body and soul.

In this chapter we will sketch the context of practices and culture around birth in Western societies. In this exploration of the importance of 'holding the space' in labour and birth there is a weaving of notions, *presence*, *consciousness* and *guardianship* in order to capture the meanings of 'being-there' as midwives. In the process of writing this chapter the meaning of words and terms became an important aspect of our sharing dialogue. It was important that these meanings were shared to bring coherence to the chapter. Table 7.1 presents our mutually agreed definitions.

Context

The literature on health and on childbirth recognises that in Western healthcare systems childbirth is viewed as a hospital and medical matter. There is a culture of technoscience, risk aversion and of surveillance creating a background hum or mood of fear. As a working environment, the hospital generates fragmented, routinised and standardised care, embodying a conveyor belt mentality in the name of performance and efficiency. The vision of care is more technical than relational and the uniqueness of each woman is usually not considered in the provision of care (Tew 1990, Davis-Floyd 1992).

In the learning environment of health sciences, the authoritative knowledge is the medical one which is learned by most undergraduate students of medicine. In the textbook *Williams Obstetrics*, considered the bible of obstetrical knowledge, we read the definition of birth as: 'The complete expulsion or extraction from the mother of a foetus after 20 weeks' gestation' (Cunningham et al. 2010, 3). This definition is a perfect example of the mechanistic and fragmented perspective on a fundamental process for human beings: being born. Childbirth as a transformative process of highly social importance is not part of the obstetrical vocabulary. Labour progress is fixed in specific phases and all obstetrics procedures/protocols are coming from (often rigid) interpretation of the measures of the woman's body and established limits of normality. What is outside those limits is usually considered as a reason to intervene (Zhang et al. 2002, Murphey-Lawless 1998).

However, the problem of technoscience is not its capacity to resolve problems of pathology but the subtle insinuation that it could 'improve' physiology. For decades, women's bodies have been constructed and perceived as defective. Traditionally, the foetus was considered to be protected by his mother. In many medical disciplines the foetus is conceived as having to be protected 'from' his mother (Rothman 2000). This biomedical model is using the positivist scientific principles which believe that 'truth' can only come from the systematic exclusion

TABLE 7.1 Our mutually agreed definitions[1]

Concepts and notions	Definitions
Space	'Space' is the invisible realm of 'place' filled with the energy of relationships (Lemay and Hastie 2016)
Quantum Physics	Explains the nature and behaviour of matter and energy on the atomic and subatomic level as interconnecting, dynamic fields of particles and waves of possibilities; the observer and the observed affect and change each other; there is no objective reality (Merches 2012)
Presence	A whole body or whole being experience of focused attention in the moment (Waterworth et al. 2015)
Complexity Theory	Refers to complex systems that are dynamic and defined more by relationships than by their constituent parts (Castellani and Hafferty 2009)
Sacred	That which has special meaning or significance to the beholder – status derived from association with particular aspects of culture and custom; anchors values and gives meaning (Lemay and Hastie 2016)
Power	Energy which enables an individual or a group to do what they want; power is essential for living; without power we are not able to move at all; power is ethically neutral (Foucault 1980).
Consciousness	• Awareness • Theories about consciousness range from the materialist to the transcendent • Materialists claim it is 'an emergent by-product of physical or computational processes' • The transcendent perspective claims it to be the ultimate reality from which physical reality emerges (Noble, Crotty and Karande 2016) • The transcendent perspective is the definition used in this chapter
Spirit	Life force, animating principle, vital spark, breath of life; 'élan vital', 'the spirit of nature' (Merriam-Webster Online Dictionary)
Spirituality	The yearning to discover the meaning and purpose of our lives (we are both meaning seekers and meaning makers); it is a vital awareness that infuses all aspects of our being; the capacity to experience wonder and a sense of connectedness (Tischler, Biberman and McKeage 2002, Mooney and Timmins 2007)
Energy	A dynamic force; power which may be translated into motion, overcoming resistance, or affecting physical change; the ability to do work (Oschman 2016)
Zero-Point Field	The quantum state with the lowest possible energy; contains fleeting electromagnetic waves and particles that pop into and out of existence (McTaggart 2003)
Quantum Zeno Effect	The evolution of a system can be 'frozen' by frequent measurements (Pradhan 2015), the 'watched pot never boils effect'

of subjectivity and that health and disease can only be explained by biochemical factors (Murphey-Lawless 1998).

The predominant methodology of research in maternity health care is epidemiology and creating a statistical based knowledge that aims at certainty. The word 'evidence' is conceived around numbers, whereas spirituality as human existential evidence is often ignored. (McGrath 1997). The Evidence Based Medicine (EBM) mindset is also adding a plethora of guidelines in all birth places which are expected to be applied. The resultant contemporary situation in and around childbirth is that thinking and acting outside this matrix is not valued by organisations that privilege a biomedical approach and complete standardisation of care. Yet in the world of 20th and 21st century science a revolution has occurred in the fields of physic quantum theory, theory of complexity and theory of chaos, bringing a new paradigm to explore and understand the reality in which we live. As Soo Downe (2008) argues simplicity and linearity are no longer sufficient to explain complex phenomenon like childbirth.

We live in a participatory universe of inherent interconnectedness. Reality is not in the substance. It is in the relation; an observer is not separated from what she/he observes. An energetic connection exists and whatever energy is brought to an encounter, conscious or not, influences the interaction. Even if complexity has entered into many disciplines, it seems that obstetrical sciences are still functioning with the values and concepts of the age of Enlightenment (simplicity, determinism, ideal of regularity and certainty). If the universe is not a big machine, neither is the human body.

We have both found that this is mirrored in childbirth and contend that childbearing is a complex dynamic adaptive system and not purely a bodily mechanical process as the biomedical model proposes. According to astrophysics, a significant part of our reality is in fact invisible. The exploration of spirituality is therefore not a solely esoteric quest; it is an experiential part of our world. To know and accept this invisible reality certainly challenges the mindset of many midwives and others who find themselves at birth.

Issues related to the domination of institutionalisation and medicalisation of childbirth are also issues concerning the domination of institutionalisation and medicalisation of midwifery practice. May be it is time to name, explore and work for a reappropriation of the midwives' paradigm. The notion of the presence of the midwife 'holding the space' is part of that journey. For the sake of this chapter those attending birth in a professional role are understood as midwives. This is not to deny that others, not professionally educated and regulated as midwives, provide midwifery support to women through childbirth.

Presence

How often have you experienced talking to someone who seemed distracted? While that person was physically present, their mind and their essence were elsewhere. How did you experience that conversation? How did you feel when you left the presence of the person? Did you feel heard or cared about? How often have you been distracted when talking with another? What message did you send? Too often, our lives are full. The proliferation of mobile devices and phones can constantly pull us away from what is in front of us. We run from activity to activity with our minds on what we haven't done yet and what we have still to do. However, humans feel valued, respected and important when the other person is fully present to us. Being present means having our attention focused 'in the moment'; fully being in the 'now' – within the present moment (Tolle 2005). When we are fully 'present', we bring our whole complex selves – physical, energetic, cultural, emotional, cognitive and spiritual – as well as our personal philosophy into resonance with the subject of our attention. Being 'present' involves a calm awareness of what is happening in our own bodies and minds as it is happening, without shifting our attentional focus.

This state of witnessing our own internal processes is 'mindfulness', an ego-less state of conscious awareness (Shapiro and Carlson 2009). Our ego can be understood as the sum total of our recurring thought forms generated by our conditioned mental emotional patterns that form our individuated sense of self (Grof 1993, Peck 1993). Tolle (2005) contends that the ego-less state of conscious awareness is our spiritual self, the ground of our being. McTaggart (2003) describes this being at-one as the 'the Zero Point Field', the essence of all that is, when we are in the 'now'. This oneness is explained by many spiritual paths by using the analogy of our connection to infinity being like the relationship of a drop of water to the ocean. When we are in the 'now', we are receptive to what is without judgement; we are alert and attuned to the other. In everyday language we say 'we are on the same wavelength'. As midwives, we need to be aware of our own internal processes, while being mindful of the people around us. In the relationships we establish with women and their families, we are privileged to witness their experiences, ideas, hopes, fears, emotions and words as they integrate the changes that are occurring for them throughout their childbearing process. Our presence can facilitate or disrupt that process of integration (Fahy et al. 2011). Our presence as birth attendants, though, is never neutral. Carl Rogers (1951) encouraged therapists to embody a person-centred approach and an attitude of unconditional positive regard in their encounters with their clients. The core assumption of the Roger's person-centred approach is that individuals have within themselves vast resources for self-understanding, growth and development. The concept of 'presence' for the therapist and the midwife is therefore congruent. Adapting the components of a therapeutic presence espoused by Geller and Greenberg (2002) to the midwifery context it is clear how they are congruent:

a   attunement with one's self
b   being unguarded, open and receptive to what is relevant or poignant at any moment in time
c   an expanded sense of awareness, spaciousness and perception
d   clear intention of fully being 'with' women to facilitate their childbearing process.

As midwives, we intend to be fully present 'with' women, yet unaware of how we come across – perhaps being too busy and too preoccupied to be truly present. Reading Penny's story, think about how midwives respond to women when they ring or present to the birth suite in labour.

PENNY'S STORY

When Penny started labouring at 2am, a week before her due date, she was sure she would see her baby shortly. She woke her partner Tony, as she had been told that second labours and births are faster than the first. She was keen to get her mother to come and look after their son, Declan, so they could go to the hospital. When they arrived at the hospital, they went straight to the birth unit, as suggested on the prenatal orientation tour. The midwife at the front desk looked up from the computer screen, scowled, and as she returned her gaze to the computer, asked grumpily 'Did you ring to say you were coming?' Penny said she had rung. She let the midwife know that this was her second baby and she didn't think it would be long. Without looking at Penny and Tony, the midwife pointed to the waiting room halfway down the corridor and told Penny and Tony to wait there for a midwife to see them. Penny glanced at Tony as they walked down to the waiting room.

What do you think Penny and Tony's reaction would have been following that interaction with the midwife? How do you think they would have been feeling? Do you think Penny and Tony would have felt as though they are in safe hands? To consider the answers to those questions, we turn to the neuroscientist Stephen Porge's (2011) Polyvagal Theory. According to his theory, humans developed a social engagement system to survive that is mediated by the vagal nerve. Because humans are physically vulnerable, we needed to learn to get along with each other. Our nervous system developed a way of 'reading' other people while in the parasympathetic mode of the autonomic nervous system. The parasympathetic mode actively inhibits the sympathetic mode of the autonomic nervous system even in new or stressful circumstances. 'Neuroception' is the term coined by Porges (2011) to describe our subconscious ability to determine safety or threat in any given circumstance. If the situation is perceived as safe, the parasympathetic nervous system remains dominant, enabling optimal physiological functioning. However, if the neuroception of the situation is that it is unsafe, the sympathetic nervous system is activated; we become hypervigilant, emotionally reactive and ready to fight or flee. If we are unable to fight or flee, our physiology will then move to a 'freeze' state. In that 'freeze' state, people can develop feelings of hopelessness, powerlessness and loss of control, all of which can lead to trauma. In the situation with Penny and Tony, the presence of the midwife at the desk was not reassuring. Their neuroception would not have been one of safety. Their physiology would have had strong sympathetic autonomic system effects. Depending on their experience of the next midwife's presence during the labour and birth, their reception by the midwife at the desk could well have set the scene and the physiological responses for the couple to emerge from this birth feeling traumatised.

Looking through the lens of Porge's Polyvagal Theory, it is easy to see how the presence of a midwife in her/his practice encounters is of spiritual, emotional and physical importance (Pembroke and Pembroke 2008). Imagine if Penny and Tony had been greeted warmly with a smile by the midwife at the desk. Imagine if the midwife had stood up, walked around the desk, introduced herself and shaken their hands. Imagine if she had welcomed them to the birth unit and let them know that they would be well looked after. Imagine if she had gone even further and asked about the other child, congratulated them on having this baby and made some kindly comment about looking forward to seeing the child. What effect do you think the warm, welcoming presence of the midwife described above would have on Penny and Tony?

We contend that mindful self-aware midwives understand that all living entities are sensitive to the energies in the environment. If we are mindful and self-aware, we know that the smile in our voice transmits over the phone and is picked up by the person on the other end. Mindful and self-aware birth attendants, whether midwives or doctors, are fully 'present' in their interactions with the women and families they serve. Being 'present' is about being conscious; that is aware of one's internal and external environment in a discerning, non-judgemental manner. Mindful, self-awareness enables the midwife/doctor to ensure their 'presence' communicates interest, kindness, respect and warmth as they understand that to do so has significant consequences.

Spiritual nature of birth

Consciousness, we contend, is an integral part of presence; it is a kind of knowledge and experience that cannot be learned. Although being and becoming conscious of something is almost an everyday experience in human life the question remains, *what* are we conscious of?

We contend that spirituality is normal; it is not something 'new' and it doesn't come only in certain places or only with physiological birth. We don't have to 'add' it to the care women and families receive. We have to remember that it is implicit to the human's 'being-in-the-world'. The context of childbirth is often demarcated into the normal and the pathological as if that is all there is. However, we need to be cautious not to assume that all medical colleagues adhere to such a defined demarcation (see Alison Barrett's chapter 'Spiritual obstetrics'). We may have hidden the existential and spiritual dimension of birth at cost. By neglecting the spiritual dimension of the experience of the woman we are also neglecting the spiritual dimension of everybody present in the place of birth. The spiritual nature of birth can be simply living our connectedness

(Burkhardt and Nagai-Jacobson 2002). Acknowledging this connectedness at birth can help everybody focus more on persons rather than on tasks alone.

In different disciplines, such as psychology, sociology and anthropology, childbirth is considered a period of adjustment and of personal and social transformation (Rich 1980, Martin 1987, Rabuzzi 1994, Bergeret-Amselek 1997, Prinds et al. 2014). Moreover, some authors consider childbirth as a spiritual emergency i.e. a transformative life experience which can lead someone to question and often change her/his values and meanings in life (Hall and Taylor in Downe 2004). While passage through this kind of condition can be difficult, sometimes traumatic and frightening, these states have tremendous healing and growth potential (Collins 2008).

Providing care at birth with a vision informed purely by the biomedical paradigm does not honour the deep significance of the event. Maybe it is the definition of birth that has to be challenged, changed and expanded. Indeed, we contend that the real problem of the biomedical knowledge is not that it is dominant but that it is insufficient, causing a poverty of culture around birth. The spiritual dimension of birth should be honoured in every birth place globally. Marcel Gauchet (1985) propounded the term 'disenchantment of the World' which can be understood as the depletion of the reign of the invisible. Can we, as birth attendants, work for the *re-enchantment* of the world starting with birth? As Jan Christilaw said when she was the president of the Society of Obstetricians and Gynaecologists of Canada (SOGC), we need to 'restore the wonder ... Birth is so precious' (personal communication 2009).

Being conscious doesn't come with an obligation of doing everything differently. However, when you are conscious, even if you do the same, nothing's the same. Being conscious of the invisible at birth can be illustrated by the following personal story of a very experienced obstetrician explaining to a resident doctor what is 'really' important (and invisible) at birth, beyond required clinical skills.

PERSONAL STORY

This head doctor obstetrician was teaching the new resident the manoeuvres for delivering a baby. They were in a cubicle with a table, a torso and a doll and the obstetrician demonstrated the movements the foetus makes to be born. After a few demonstrations, the obstetrician said to the resident that it was time for him to be exposed to a 'real' birth; that they would find a woman who was pushing and that he, the resident, would be in charge. When they arrived at the door of a woman in second stage of labour, the obstetrician turned to the young resident and said, 'You know what? What I just taught you, forget it. When you enter in a birthing room, you first have to be able to see the angels that are present in the space. You know, it took me at least ten years to be able to be really conscious of that ...

Making meaning and seeking meaning

During an archaeological dig archaeologists found a variety of artefacts including graves with tools, traces of rituals and symbols related to death. From these finds the archaeologists concluded that human beings had lived there. What can be understood here is that we are not human because of our mammal biology and physicochemical components. A body is human because it is inscribed in a symbolic order. Human beings are making and seeking meaning and longing for connections. Likewise, birth is not just a hormonal and biological process that has to be safely supported and facilitated; it is an event with great significance in human life. The following story of an Inuit remote community of Canada illustrates how giving meaning is vital to the life of any human being.

PERSONAL STORY

For many years, the people in the small village (800 inhabitants) of Salluit in the North of Québec (Nunavik) had been making moves to bring birth back in their community. They wanted a birthing centre in the village and also Inuit midwives to serve women and families. During previous decades, pregnant women were evacuated by plane to a place six to eight hours away in the south (Montreal) three weeks before their due date and returned three weeks after the birth. Families were split apart with deep social consequences. In the autumn of 2004, a meeting of community members and health care providers from the South was held to discuss the project. At the meeting, women explained that it is important and normal to 'give life' in their own village. The professionals talked about 'safety' and explained the dangers of giving birth so far from a hospital and from a caesarean section if needed.

One of the elders, who had been sitting quietly, listening to all the comments said: 'I can understand that some of you may think that birth in remote areas is dangerous. We have made it clear what it means for our women to birth in our community. And you really must know that a life without meaning is much more dangerous.'

Another story highlights the capacity to go beyond fear and risk that is often culturally linked to birth.

THE YOUNG FATHER'S STORY

A young father and his partner planned to give birth to their first baby at home with a midwife. Labour was so fast that the baby arrived before the midwife arrived and the parents were alone at home. The midwife arrived at the moment of the placenta being born. A few weeks after the birth, at the last postnatal visit with the midwife, the father gave her a card. He had written: 'There are some mornings where you feel like you're at the dawn of the Universe.'

The young father expressed clearly his consciousness of the immense and almost cosmic dimension of birth. We can understand that being conscious of the spiritual nature of birth and taking this into account is about being fully human. This speaks of the need to humanise birth.

Humanising birth

Concerns on the humanisation of health care have been growing worldwide. There was an International Conference on Humanization of Childbirth held in Brazil in 2000. The conference brought together close to 2,000 participants from more than 23 countries, including representatives from UNICEF and WHO. Affirming the importance of starting at birth, the following definition of humanisation was adopted:

> A process of communication and caring between people leading to self-transformation and an understanding of the fundamental spirit of life and a sense of compassion for and unity with: the Universe, the spirit and nature; other people in the family, the community, the country and global society; and other people in future, as well as past generations. ... humanisation can be applied to any aspect of care, including childbirth. As childbirth is the beginning of life and affects the rest of life, and because the humanisation of childbirth is such a clear need, the application of this particular aspect of care is an important start.
>
> *(Umenai et al. 2001, S3–4)*

It is interesting to note that nowhere do the terms 'spirituality' or 'spiritual' appear in this definition. Yet, it is *everywhere* and *implicit*; it is light years on from the usual idea of gentleness associated with the notion of humanisation. We would contend that spirituality is not 'out there'; it is 'in there', 'within' each of us. We do not need to add something to what we already do. We mainly have to *remember* that spirituality is a fundamental and normal part of human's being-in-the-world and evidence of our existential interconnected humanness. When we become conscious of the deep meaning of humanisation it reveals to us how birth belongs to humanity as a spiritual event. In understanding this we see how compassion and kindness are essential in the care around birth and how guardianship of birth is crucial.

Midwifery Guardianship

Midwifery Guardianship (Fahy and Hastie 2008) is a sub-concept of Birth Territory Theory (Fahy et al. 2011). The concept of 'birth territory' is defined as everything external to the woman. Everything external to the woman is conceptualised as encompassing all elements of the environment from the micro level of the individual birth space, to the political, historical, legal, professional and regulatory frameworks that control what is possible at the micro level.

Birth Territory Theory can be used to describe, explain and predict how the environment – the 'birth territory' – affects women, babies and midwives in terms of both process and outcomes (Fahy et al. 2011).

We contend that the midwife's presence as described by Pembroke and Pembroke (2008) is a key part of a woman's birth territory. 'Midwifery Guardianship' is a term used to conceptualise that presence as a mindful one that is aware of and utilises her/his inner power to connect with the woman while creating and maintaining harmony within the woman's birth territory (Fahy and Hastie 2008). Inner power is 'spirit' – that omnipresent electromagnetic life-force that is part of universal energy. Like universal energy, our inner power is ethically neutral. Midwives and others can use their inner power in an integrative or disintegrative manner (Fahy and Hastie 2008). When Integrative Power is operational, all power within the birthing environment is focused on supporting the woman to feel safe and let go of her everyday thinking mind (Hastie 2008). When a labouring woman feels safe, she is enabled to enter a state of non-ordinary consciousness (Fahy and Hastie 2008). In this state of non-ordinary consciousness, a woman's mind-body-spirit is integrated and she can sense and spontaneously respond to her intuitions, body's signals and its changes throughout the birthing process (see also Chapter 8 by Jenny Parratt). Whereas the use of Integrative Power is facilitative, the use of Disintegrative Power is disruptive, fragmenting the birthing woman's mind-body-spirit and weakening her energy. Disintegrative Power is associated with the imposition of someone's self-serving goal. The effect is a disintegration of the power held by other people in the birth room (Fahy and Hastie 2008). Disintegrative Power can be used by the woman, midwife or others in the birth territory determined to have a specific experience or outcome. Regardless of who uses Disintegrative Power, the woman's capacity to feel, trust and respond spontaneously to her bodily sensations and intuitions is undermined (Fahy and Hastie 2008).

If you think back to the situation with Penny and Tony and the behaviour of the midwife at the reception desk, do you think the midwife was using her inner power in an integrative or disintegrative way? Was that midwife seeking to create and maintain harmony in Penny's birth territory? The converse of Midwifery Guardianship is Midwifery Domination. When a midwife is seeking to dominate the situation for her own goals, whether consciously or unconsciously, she is using her inner power in an egoic manner. A midwife who is 'present' and mindfully practicing the principles of Midwifery Guardianship is calm, alert and attuned to the power dynamics in the birth room. As she/he attunes to the woman and is on the same wavelength, 'messages' such as subtle body changes perceived as 'intuitive feelings' and/or words can be telepathically received, much like a radio station when we are tuned to its particular frequency. In this way the midwife can sense and become aware that the woman needs to change position or is feeling frightened or that someone in the room is getting impatient and wants the labour to hurry up, without any words being spoken. The following personal story (Carolyn) highlights the importance of attuning in the right way:

PERSONAL STORY

Angela, a Chinese woman, was in labour with her third baby. Her mother-in-law and sister-in-law were in the birthing room with her. The midwife had already talked with Angela about the fact that both the other women seemed to be distracting Angela from the labour. Angela had said that she'd rather have a longer labour than ask them to leave because she would pay for it forever. Several hours later, Angela was standing, rocking backwards and forwards, one leg up on a chair and groaning loudly. The midwife sensed that the baby was ready to be born and Angela was holding back. The midwife asked Angela what she was thinking. Angela said she was thinking 'I can't do it', that 'it's too hard'. The midwife asked her 'What's the other half of you thinking?' Angela glanced at the midwife with a shocked expression on her face, as though she'd been 'caught out' and murmured 'I want to have this baby now it's ready to be born'. The midwife whispered 'Why don't you ask that part of you to join the other part of you and decide to have this baby together?' Angela paused for a while, closed her eyes and breathed deeply for several minutes. When the next wave of uterine activity came, Angela flashed a smile at the midwife and said 'I can do it, baby is coming' and her baby was born easily and well with that contraction. The placenta followed soon after.

By attuning in this way the Midwifery Guardianship quality in Angela's story reflects a midwife's deep awareness and respect of the ancient genetic program for childbearing and birthing encoded in every woman's DNA. The midwife is at once present and conscious to the myriad possibilities that can play out in Angela's individual experience. Angela's long labour provides an opportunity to consider the Quantum Zeno Effect.

Quantum Zeno informs us that when particles are moving towards a resolution, frequent measurements freeze the action in time, inhibiting progress (Pradhan 2015). While particle physics are not yet applied to the human being, we argue they should be because humans are a mass of particles and various quantum physics phenomena. The Quantum Zeno Effect could explain a lot of what we see at birth. The impatient surveillance exhibited by Angela's in-laws can be theorised to have provided that freezing effect on Angela's labour progression. It was only when Angela chose to change what she was thinking that her baby was born. In this way the Midwifery Guardian in Angela's story seeks to 'hold the space'.

That 'space' is the Zero Point Field of possibilities. When a midwife uses her/his power to act to create or restore the focus of everyone in the 'space' to the shared higher goal of supporting the woman's sacred work of birthing new life, she/he facilitates an environment where the woman feels safe, supported and free to relax into the birthing process.

Holding the space: being a guardian

The notion of 'holding the space' is probably not new in the literature but it was one of the most significant themes of my (Céline) doctoral research that examined the lived experience of practising midwives in the 1980s in Québec, Canada (Lemay 2007). The exploration of the theme will be explored here further, bringing new insights to our representation of birth. (Note: The following quotes are free translations from French texts).

For the midwives interviewed, 'holding the space' was not related to a place or territory, to an action or to a particular kind of birth. For Rachel it was like being 'a lighted lamp, a conscious presence'. For Alice the space was essentially a 'space of recognition' where the sacred and mysterious character of birth was recognised. She felt that she had the responsibility to protect this space, wherever the place of birth, to make sure that it will not be trampled.

The meanings and significance of 'holding the space' for the midwives in that research were closely linked to a sense of guardianship. What is interesting is my findings were not so much about 'where' and 'how' to hold the space, but more about '*why*' doing it and being a guardian of the space was significant. The midwives in my study had three profound representations of pregnancy and childbirth: a space of possibilities, a space of mystery and a space of passages. I will highlight each in turn.

Birth as a space of possibilities

Like other unfolding life processes, everything in childbirth is possible. Life will come but nothing is guaranteed; nothing is absolutely certain. Because childbirth is a space of possibilities, midwives in the study considered themselves as guardians of this open and undetermined space. The midwives 'don't know' *exactly* what will happen and paradoxically they found that kind of 'non-knowledge' important. When the obstetrical culture is considering mostly the possibilities of complications, the midwives were considering childbirth as possibilities and transformations: self-discovery, healing, courage, self-opening, miracle, accomplishment, etc. When some are seeing risks, the midwives in the study were seeing 'occasions' of potentiality. Midwives were there to help women to accomplish their potential (whatever it can be) because the experience of giving birth can be a source of personal power. Childbirth can change a woman so she can relate to her child and change her entire way of being-in-the-world.

Birth is not a matter of success/failure or performance. A woman can be helped to honour her own process where she is able to mobilise her own inner strengths whatever the circumstances of her birth. Although medicine may see birth as a situation through the lens of risk, midwives in my study viewed birth as a special transformative and empowering occasion for women.

Birth can be an occasion full of possibilities for a woman revealing 'power from within her' not a 'power over her'. Experiencing such power from within can be a stepping stone towards autonomy and self-affirmation in a woman's life. My study highlighted the moment of birth where confidence and fear, anguish and joy, power and fragility emerged. Space and time at birth is a deep part of who we are (see Chapter 2 by Susan Crowther). For Anne, the discovery of this space was akin to something sacred:

> When a woman is giving birth she is also giving birth to herself, again and again and this discovery is an important part of the process.
>
> *(Lemay 2007, 159)*

Anne's presence at birth was to 'protect and nourish' what was about to be born, being conscious that in that space not only a baby was born.

Pregnancy, like a seed, a chrysalis, or an egg, is a promise, the promise of a child, a flower, a butterfly or a bird. The possibilities of a new life are strong yet also fragile because nothing can guarantee that the promises will be kept. Fortunately midwives have the repeated experience of kept promises. This is what makes them confident and joyful. Yet, like all birth attendants, they have the experience of unkept promises around birth. The unpredictability of birth calls for humility and not thinking of ourselves as *the* guardian of life. For midwives, uncertainty *is* the field where all possibilities are in constant movement. Lévesque (1976, 27) says: 'Nothing is more effective and subversive than a simple possibility.' This is no less true at each birth.

Birth as a space of mystery

Birth is not just a space of possibilities. Being there and holding the space is giving to the midwife a 'gaze' that enables her to 'see' beyond the practical and clinical aspects of her practice. As Anne says: 'There is so much more in life than what we just see' (Lemay 2007, 162). Childbirth is often described as a moment where something huge and powerful in presence. We see words like 'miracle' 'mystery', 'wonder' and 'oceanic feeling' (Joël 2002, Kahn 1995, Cosslet 1994, Rossi 2002/3) in different studies. Birth seems to create a sense of awe and is an encounter with the numinous, a mystery we will never fully understand. In a world of transformations, midwives in my study found themselves at the interface between visible and invisible realities. The visible is arguably obvious and important. Yet, a midwife declares, 'It is not that. It is greater than that. It is more than that. It is greater than us' (Lemay 2007, 165). I would contend that midwives are guardians of this 'greater than that'. There is a sacred character of birth beyond specific religious and secular beliefs, as Alice (midwife) explains:

> If I say the sacred moment of birth, I know that many parents don't see the sacred moment of birth. It is not less sacred. I hold this space in the place of birth. I have to keep it consciously alive inside me.
>
> *(Lemay 2007, 166)*

The sacred dimension of birth is the connection to the mysteries of the world and of life. For Elizabeth (midwife) this space is like a gift that deserves protection:

> [I]t brings us deeper into the meaning and the connection that you have in life ... if we are becoming conscious of the depth of what we live perhaps it can make us more awake to the beauty that is around us, and maybe we would protect it.
>
> *(Lemay 2007, 166)*

Birth as a space of passages

Davis-Floyd (1992) and Reed, Barnes and Rowe (2016) view birth as a major life passage. For women this major life passage lies at the heart of all social groups – a process of emergence that has a high initiatory value as it is acknowledged and accompanied by specific and traditional rituals.

Midwives in my study considered themselves as guardians of the passages of childbirth, respecting, honouring, sometimes helping and often protecting the processes. It gave a special meaning to their presence during childbirth. Birth as a space of passages opens a time where we are most aware of our connections and of being mutually fragile. What is said, done, wherever and however the birth unfolds is significant. As Maryse explains:

> This is midwifery. A present energy to the woman and the child in order to enable a sacred passage. I was there for that.
>
> *(Lemay 2007, 168)*

For midwives in my study being-there at a birth is very much about learning to inhabit the space of birth, a background or matrix space where we experience the infinite *in* the finite and the eternal connections *between* the visible and invisible of the lifeworld (*Lebenswelt*). When we become conscious of this depth of reality we realise that birth has a highly spiritual dimension and that being a birth attendant cannot be reduced exclusively to the physical presence and the provision of clinical care and safety.

By exploring the notion of 'holding the space' at birth as a space of possibilities, a space of mystery and a space of passages we come to understand the spiritual dimension of midwifery practice and appreciate how closely this relates to midwifery guardianship.

Conclusion

In this chapter, our goal has been to encourage you, the reader, to consider the sacred nature of the work in being a midwife and 'holding space' for a childbearing woman in her ever-changing process of transformation that comes with bringing new life into the world. Our perspective is a *pragmatic spirituality* in that we suggest the whole of life is spiritual, as much as it is physical, if not more so. We contend that everything starts in spirit, also known as the Zero Point Field, and manifests into form according to our orientation; our philosophy, values and beliefs; our intention, our worldview and awareness; our consciousness; our previous experiences; and our vision. To us as experienced midwives from two very different regions on Earth, spirituality is not only esoteric; it is an integral part of being human allowing new ways of knowing while trusting in the intelligence of our lived complexity. As birth attendants we are privileged to be invited into the special moments of others' lives. During those moments we don't need to 'do' more; our quest is to 'be' more – more self and other aware; more open; kinder; more compassionate; more conscious while silencing the technological imperative to constantly 'do'.

Note

1 All 'Lemay and Hastie 2016' references are through our conversations during our time writing this chapter.

References

Bergeret-Amselek A. 1997. *Le Mystère des Mères*. Paris: Desclée de Brouwer.

Burkhardt M.A. and Nagai-Jacobson M.G. 2002. *Spirituality: Living our connectedness*. Australia: Delmar, Thomson Learning.

Carrier, M. 2005. *Penser le sacré. Les sciences humaines et l'invention du sacré*. Montréal: Liber.

Castellani, B. and Hafferty, F. 2009. *Sociology and complexity science*. Heidelberg: Springer.

Collins, M. 2008. 'Spiritual emergency: transpersonal, personal, and political dimensions.' *Psychotherapy and Politics International*, 6(1): 3–16. doi:10.1002/ppi.147.

Cosslett, T. 1994. *Women writing childbirth*. New York: Manchester University Press.

Cunningham F.G. et al. 2010. *Williams Obstetrics*, 23rd edn. New York: McGraw Hill Medical.

Davis-Floyd, R.E. 1992. *Birth as an American rite of passage*. Berkeley, CA: University of California Press.

Dean K. 2004. 'The role of methods in maintaining orthodox beliefs in health research.' *Social Science & Medicine*, 58: 675–685.

Downe, S. 2008. *Normal Childbirth. Evidence and Debate*. London: Churchill Livingstone.

Fahy, K. and Hastie, C, 2008. Midwifery Guardianship: Reclaiming the sacred in birth. In K. Fahy, M. Foureur and C. Hastie (eds), *Birth territory and midwifery guardianship: Theory for practice, education and research* (pp. 21–37). Edinburgh: Elsevier.

Fahy, K., Parratt, J., Foureur, M. and Hastie, C. 2011. Birth territory: A theory for midwifery practice. In R. Bryar and M. Sinclair (eds), *Theory for midwifery practice*, 2nd edn (pp. 215–240). Palgrave: Basingstoke.

Foucault, M. 1980. *Power/Knowledge: Selected interviews*. New York: Pantheon.

Gauchet, M. 1985. *Le désenchantement du monde*. Paris: Gallimard.

Geller, S. M. and Greenberg, L.S. 2002. 'Therapeutic Presence: Therapists' experience of presence in the psychotherapy encounter / Therapeutische Präsenz: Erfahrungen von Therapeuten mit Präsenz in der psychotherapeutischen Begegnung / La Presencia Terapéutica: La Experiencia de la Presencia que Viven los Terapeutas en el Encuentro Psicoterapéutico.' *Person-Centered & Experiential Psychotherapies* 1(1–2): 71–86. doi:10.1080/14779757.2002.9688279

Grof, C. 1993. *The thirst for wholeness: Attachment, addiction and the spiritual path.* San Francisco, CA: HarperCollins.

Hall, J. 2010. Spirituality and labour care. In D. Walsh and S. Downe (eds), *Essential midwifery practice: Intrapartum care* (pp. 235–251). London: Blackwell Publishing Ltd.

Hall, J. and Taylor, M. 2004. Birth and spirituality. In S. Downe (ed.) *Normal Childbirth: Evidence and Debate* (pp. 41–56). London: Churchill Livingstone.

Hastie, C. 2008. *Putting women first: Interprofessional integrative power.* (Master of Philosophy), University of Newcastle, Newcastle. Retrieved from http://hdl.handle.net/1959.13/29305.

Joël, M. 2002. *Enfantement, allaitement, féminisme.* Retreived from http://joel.martine.free.fr

Jordan B. 1993. *Birth in four cultures: A crosscultural investigation of childbirth in Yucatan, Holland, Sweden, and the United States.* Prospect Heights, IL: Waveland Press.

Kahn, R.P. 1995. *Bearing meaning: the language of birth.* Urbana, IL: University of Illinois Press.

Lemay, C. 2007. "Être là": étude du phénomène de la pratique sage-femme au Québec dans les années 1970–1980, PhD thesis (unpublished), Applied Human Sciences, University of Montreal.

Lévesque, C. 1976. *L'étrangeté du texte.* Québec: VLB.

Marchand, L. 2015. 'Shared presence: The heart of the therapeutic relationship.' *Families, Systems & Health*, 33(3): 283.

Martin E. 1987. *The woman in the body: A cultural analysis of reproduction.* Boston, MA: Beacon Press.

McGrath, P. 1997 'Putting the spirituality on the agenda: Hospice research findings on the "ignored Dimension".' *Hospice Journal*, 12(4): 1–14.

McTaggart, L. 2003. *The Field*, 2nd edn. New York: Harper Collins.

Merches, I. 2012. *Basics of quantum electrodynamics.* Hoboken, NJ: CRC Press.

Merriam-Webster Online Dictionary, accessed 10 June 2016 www.merriam-webster.com/dictionary/spirit.

Morin, E. 1990. *Introduction à la pensée complexe.* Paris: E.S.F.

Mooney, B. and Timmins, F. 2007. 'Spirituality as a universal concept: Student experience of learning about spirituality through the medium of art.' *Nurse Education in Practice*, 7(5): 275–284. http://doi.org/10.1016/j.nepr.2006.09.001.

Murphey-Lawless J. 1998. *Reading birth and death: A history of obstetric thinking.* Indianapolis, IN: Indiana University Press.

Noble, K.D., Crotty, J.J. and Karande, A. 2016. 'Why consciousness? Teaching and learning at the leading edge of mind science.' *NeuroQuantology*, 14(2): 175–192.

Oschman, J.L. 2016. *Energy medicine: The scientific basis*, 2nd edn. London: Elsevier.

Peck, M.S. 1993. *The road less travelled: A new psychology of love, traditional values and spiritual growth.* London: Hutchinson.

Pembroke, N.F. and Pembroke, J.J. 2008. 'The spirituality of presence in midwifery care.' *Midwifery*, 24(3): 321–327. doi:http://dx.doi.org/10.1016/j.midw.2006.10.004.

Porges, S.W. 2011. *The Polyvagal Theory.* New York: W.W. Norton & Company.

Pradhan, R.K. 2015. 'Quantum Zeno Effect in sleep disorders and treatment by the anti-zeno effect.' *NeuroQuantology*, 14(1): 143–148. http://doi.org/10.14704/nq.2016.14.1.864.

Prinds, C., Hvidt, N.C., Mogensen, O. and Buus, N. 2014. 'Making existential meaning in transition to motherhood: A scoping review.' *Midwifery*, 30(6): 733–741.

Rabuzzi, KA. 1994. *Mother with child: Transformation through childbirth.* Indianapolis, IN: Indiana University Press.

Reed, R., Barnes, M. and Rowe, J. 2016. 'Women's experience of birth: Childbirth as a rite of passage.' *International Journal of Childbirth*, 6(1): 46–56.

Rich, A. 1980. *Naître d'une femme, la maternité en tant qu'expérience et institution*. Paris: Denoël-Gonthier.

Rogers, C. 1951. *Client-centered therapy: Its current practice, implications and theory*. London: Constable.

Rossi, P. 2002/3 'Eclosion du matriciel, expérience du féminin.' *Dialogue*, no. 157: 51–58.

Rothman, B.K. 2000. *Recreating motherhood: Ideology and technology in a patriarchal society*, 2nd edn. New Brunswick, NJ: Rutgers University Press.

Shapiro, S. L. and Carlson, L.E. 2009. *The art and science of mindfulness*. Washington, DC: American Psychological Association.

Tew, M. 1990. *Safer childbirth?: A critical history of maternity care*. London: Chapman and Hall.

Tischler, T., Biberman, J. and McKeage, R. 2002. 'Linking emotional intelligence, spirituality and workplace performance: Definitions, models and ideas for research.' *Journal of Managerial Psychology*, 17 (3): 203–218. doi: 10.1108/02683940210423114.

Tolle, E. 2005. *The power of now: A guide to spiritual enlightenment*, 2nd edn. San Francisco, CA: New World Library.

Umenai T., Wagner M., et al. 2001. 'Conference agreement on the definition of humanization and humanized care.' *International Journal of Gynecology and Obstetrics*, 75(2001): S3–S4.

Waterworth, J.A., Waterworth, E.L., Riva, G. and Mantovani, F. 2015. Presence: Form, content and consciousness. In M. Lombard, F. Biocca, J. Freeman, W. Ijsselsteijn, and J.R. Schaevitz (eds), *Immersed in media: Telepresence theory, measurement & technology* (pp. 35–58). Cham, Switzerland: Springer International Publishing.

Zhang, J., Troendle, J.F. and Yancey, M.K. 2002. 'Reassessing the labor curve in nulliparous women.' *American Journal of Obstetrics & Gynecology*, 187(4): 824–828.

8

COUPLES' SPIRITUAL EXPERIENCES AT BIRTH

Jenny Parratt

At the last birth I attended, the woman stood powerfully in a birth pool while she and her partner guided their baby into the world. Together, they held the baby and marvelled at their achievement. The joy and sense of connection between this couple and their baby was palpably obvious to all who were present. Throughout the previous few hours this woman and her partner had laboured individually and together through the various challenges they had been presented with. The woman had responded to each strengthening contraction with various movements and sounds; her partner had moved with her, massaging and providing physical support. She 'zoned out', dropping into a progressively deeper altered conscious state while her partner, who knew her mannerisms and sounds so well, acted as an intermediary to ensure the birth environment was meeting her needs. This couple had already formed a relationship with their birth attendants who were each willing guides: their attendants acted respectfully with the couple and used their knowledge to ensure any issues were addressed according to the couple's particular needs. The couple felt both safe enough and empowered to steer their own course toward the miracle of their baby's birth. I felt that a special space had opened, a space that I name spiritual. In this spiritual space the couple appeared to experience the power of their own capability as it dissolved any fears of the present and the future. The reward for each of us present on that day was to share the joy of spiritual experience. For me, the beauty and wonder of this birth stands in stark contrast to the first birth I attended in which this quality of spiritual space remained absent.

Sadly, I remember that first birth because it lacked any sense of what I now think of as a spiritual experience. The year was 1979 and I was a student nurse. I entered a labour room to see a woman, legs in stirrups, working hard to push her baby out. She was surrounded by people in surgical scrubs; at the end of the bed was a cajoling doctor about to apply forceps. Immediately after the birth all who were present seemed disconnected from the momentous nature of the experience. The mood was perceptibly flat and genuine interaction between anyone in the room was absent. Although the result was a living baby, the steps to that point seemed to utterly lack vitality: (1) the woman submitted to the procedures; (2) the baby was put in her arms; and (3) she and her partner observed the baby without obvious emotion. I was shuffled out of that room, a novice puzzled by the lack of celebration for new life. Later I learnt that the sombre, robotic-like responses of doctor and midwives were in part due to their suspicion that the baby had a genetic defect.

To me, the powerful sense of achievement and wonder that can come with spiritual experiences at birth should be honoured regardless of life's imperfections. Indeed, I now know that spiritual experiences can include feelings of being whole and capable which can then positively influence how the woman and her partner experience labour, birth and parenting. Comparing the two examples above begins to illustrate how spiritual experiences are linked to and can form from a person's relationships with other people. In the first example the birth attendants worked to integrate their assessments and responses with the particular context of the couple so that both the woman and her partner could feel safe and empowered. In contrast, the second example showed attendants who disengaged from a couple who appeared to be powerless. Honouring that couple's experience would instead have required the attendants to not only hold and act on concerns for the baby but also to respectfully engage with the couple. Consider for a moment how this second couple might more positively have approached parenting if they had been enabled toward spiritual experiences during labour and birth.

The focus of this chapter is on spiritual experiences, relationality and childbirth. When considering relationality, I focus on three key people: the labouring woman; her partner in labour; and the midwife. A woman's partner in labour may be of any gender; this person may be her intimate partner or a significant other person such as a sister. In writing this chapter I draw from my research about women's experiences of childbirth and their changing embodied sense of self (Parratt 2010, 2000). As outlined below, that research has informed the way I have approached writing this chapter and the way the key terms are defined. The research data was published as a collection of stories; I draw on these, referring to participants using pseudonyms (Parratt 2009). Other publications are drawn on too, including Valmai McDonald's conversations with parents (1992) and David Vernon's collections of stories about birth by women (2005) and by men (2006).

My approach in the chapter is similar to that in my research: feminist and post-structural. The feminist approach allows me to focus on empowering relational experiences of women and their partners (regardless of gender) and how these may be enabled (Harrison and Fahy 2005). A post-structural approach helps me to challenge 'either/or' perspectives and power imbalances (Weedon 1997). With such an approach I can take a more 'both/and' example, rather than limiting my thinking to the standard rational/irrational dichotomy, I also consider the nonrational view that is inclusive of the beauty and inexpressible wonder of spiritual experiences (Parratt and Fahy 2008). As a midwife, I add the holistic perspective so as to understand people as 'embodied selves' and define the 'embodied self' as a complex integration of body, soul and mind continually changing in relation to other people and their lived situation (Irigaray 1993, Grosz 2004, Lacan 1977, Leder 1990, Kovel 1991).

Spirituality and spirit as embodied

I define spirituality as the ways that people take to become aware of spirit and soul in their lives (Parratt 2010). Spirit in this context is the vital energy that enlivens each of us as embodied beings. Thus, the idea that people are embodied selves is an expression of how spirituality can take bodily form. For example, language honours the animating place of spirit with words such as 'respiration'; it is as if spirit enters our bodies with each breath (Parratt and Fahy 2008). Fundamentally, spirit is power; it is the nonrational, idiosyncratic, paradoxical and ethically neutral power that makes up all that is known and all that has not even begun to be imagined (Kovel 1991, Tzu 1963, Wilhelm and Baynes 1967). This understanding is in line with the concept of spirit as Universal Energy, or qi (said 'chee'; Chen 2004). A person's soul is their own uniquely embodied expression of the power of spirit; it encompasses the individual breadth and depth of what has been, what is being and what could be (Kovel 1991). Spirit and soul are expressed using power that is intrinsic to the embodied self: this I name 'intrinsic power'. Spiritual experiences, however, are limited by cultural powers – such as the pressure to conform. Similarly, a person might use the power of their ego, such as their fears or expectations, to place rational limitations on their ways of being with, and being aware of, their soul. Spiritual experiences can act as intrinsically powerful windows to the soul; either empowered or disempowered by the ways a person relates with other people and their world.

Relationality

Relationality refers to how a person's sense of who they are in the world – their being – is continually being shaped by their connections with other people (Jordan 1991, Irigaray 1996, Merleau-Ponty 2002). An integral aspect of all of life experience is that it occurs within a context of being attentive and responsive to other people (Surrey 1991). During any relational interaction, a two-way back and forth action occurs that prompts subtle changes within each person and in their sense of connection with each other. Such changes might feel empowering, or they might feel disempowering. Disempowering interactions use egoic power; this is an ego-centred power that is, for example, defensive, manipulating, dominating or submissive (Parratt 2010, Fahy et al. 2011). These interactions are disintegrative; they undermine a person's sense of connection with others and can diminish access to intrinsic power. In contrast, empowering interactions are integrative and inspiring; they involve an ongoing awareness of, and effortful negotiation with, the other person as well as with one's own egoic fears and expectations (Irigaray 2002, Parratt 2010). During these interactions there is an openness to the individual differences of the other person that convey the sense that needs and wishes are being respected and not violated (Heron 1992, Kovel 1991). Inherent in these integrative interactions is the potential of a shared joy and power which, when experienced during childbirth, can have a profound impact on how birth unfolds.

Genius birth

When a childbearing woman's relational experiences are empowering, she is more likely to have spiritual experiences and be aware of intrinsic power. Being in a spiritual experience during labour reveals the possibility of using intrinsic power to actively, effortfully and responsively participate in the birth process. A woman's full and active participation in labour can result in what I call a 'genius birth', where she gives birth according to her own particular holistic needs at that particular moment of her life (Parratt 2010, Fahy et al. 2011, Parratt 2008). In being holistically responsive to her needs, the woman draws from her whole embodied self – that complex integration of body, soul and mind at that moment.

A genius birth is usually an exceptionally powerful moment: a profound spiritual experience that is relationally meaningful and personally sacred to the woman. In the following sections, I describe how spiritual experiences are different from the rationality of ordinary experience. I then outline the ways spiritual experiences can be part of labour and I consider the impact of interactions between the woman, her partner and the midwife on such experiences. Lastly, I explain empowering ways that women, partners and others can 'be' during childbirth that enable spiritual experiences and honour birth as sacred.

Spiritual experiences: 'nonordinary' and 'nonrational'

Spiritual experiences are different from ordinary lived experience. Awareness changes during spiritual experiences making them a type of nonordinary conscious state. Consciousness occurs across a continuum from ordinary levels of every day functioning, through shallow states such as daydreaming, to deeper nonordinary states where consciousness is more profoundly altered as in during very deep meditation (Taylor 1995). The experience might be a moment embedded in the ordinariness of life, such as when watching a spectacular sunset, being hugged by a child, or breathing in the scent of a rain-washed forest. Consider for yourself: think of a time when you have felt particularly moved by life – an awesome, exhilarating moment. These experiences might be intimate, personal, or even nonsensical; nonetheless, it is their difference from what is ordinary that is likely to make them memorable and perhaps help to bring a sense of meaning to life. Late in her first pregnancy Leanne remembered such an experience with her partner:

> We lay together in the extreme silence of the Lake Eyre salt pan watching the sunrise glow a magnificent orange on the white of the salt thinking, 'we were meant to experience this.' That day was a complete reminder to enjoy today not tomorrow; it's ... easy to go to work every day counting down to Friday ... focused toward your weekend. Since starting maternity leave I've had similar sorts of overwhelming feelings of living for today.
>
> *(Parratt 2009, 131–132)*

A further aspect of spiritual experiences is that ordinary rational awareness of time and/or space are likely to alter so that perception moves beyond usual sensory boundaries of body and time (Grof 1988, Davis 1989). Perceptions of timelessness, of expansion beyond the place or person, or a sense of narrowing into the self or situation can occur. Jan Dooley said of her birth '[T]ime is a funny thing when you're labouring, it moves forward but you have no idea where it goes' (1993, 3). In the following examples Elizabeth's perception of her immediate environment altered, whereas a spatial shift was part of Sheila's experience:

> I had vivid perception. When the midwife came in she'd obviously been smoking ... the doctor had a rash on his arms ... there was a cockroach in the corner – it looked a lot bigger than it was. I remember that strange change of perception.
>
> *(Elizabeth in McDonald 1992, 5)*

> I knew I was far away. I was really in my body in that sense of being far away. The noises I was making. Every now and then I'd hear this noise. It was just so bovine, like I was a big cow.
>
> *(Sheila in McDonald 1992, 120)*

Spiritual experiences are also different because they do not fit within rational understandings of the world. Rather than being irrational though, spiritual experiences are more correctly called 'nonrational', meaning they are experientially real parts of living that are ungraspable using purely rational perspectives (Kovel 1991, 232; Parratt and Fahy 2008). This lack of fit with rational understandings occurs because spiritual experiences frequently include some sense of relational wholeness or unity. A description of the whole of something must take an inclusive 'both/and' approach rather than the usual rational contrasts of 'either this or that'; contradiction or paradox are therefore often used. The idea that Sheila (above) was both 'really in' her body, but also 'far away' is certainly a spatial paradox; her mention of being both close and far in the same sentence illustrates her nonrational sense of unity in the spatial realm. Another common way to express this relational unity experientially is through felt emotion as Stephan shows:

> I heard the baby's cry and how sweet it was. In one sense it was strong and loud but at the same time so soft and fragile. Then came the message ... 'it's a little boy!' ... I thought to myself 'Okay Stephan, you can cry for happiness,' but I simply couldn't and didn't know why ... I was so happy and so proud to be finally ... called a dad ... what a moment. It is so hard to explain or put into writing.
>
> *(Vernon 2006, 37)*

The alteration in awareness during spiritual experiences means that these experiences are also moments of relational change. Such experiential changes may merely be alterations of temporal or spatial perception, they may involve a changed awareness of the self as being intrinsically powerful, or there may be a changed sense of connection with others. At its simplest, change is an experience of being or becoming different (Parratt 2010). Stephan is essentially describing the moment that he sees himself as having now become a parent. Change can be understood in these broad terms of transition to parenthood; however, my focus in this chapter is the actual experience of being in the moments of change that are labour and birth. Later I look at the impact that partners can have in 'being there' at this time. First, I consider the woman experiencing the differentness of spiritual experience while being 'in the moment' of change that is labour.

Being in the moment of spiritual experience during labour

'Being in the moment' expresses the idea of existing in the here and now; it refers to how a person can just get on with living and put aside their thoughts or worries about the past, present and future. This is an understanding that trusts the living body as perceptive and affective as well as holding of knowing and power (Merleau-Ponty 2002). Living bodies generally know how to get on with the process of being alive without requiring too much conscious thought by the person. Sensations such as thirst, tiredness or labour pain do, however, bring bodily awareness to the forefront of one's thoughts (Leder 1990). The change in awareness that comes with spiritual experiences is part of the process that enables women to be in the moment during labour. Sometimes this change in awareness is simply a shift in focus toward moment-to-moment existence; at other times the woman might be in a deeply altered nonordinary conscious state. Jane describes her spiritual experience of what she calls 'the zone' and how she perceived herself as existing in the moment:

> I started to go into the zone when the contractions became closer together and more intense ... It's not ... something I could have prepared for but it wasn't scary, the hormones took over and I had the feeling that all that

existed was this pain and me, nothing else. When they became really intense I had that feeling that death could come and it didn't matter. It was very much just being alive in that moment and dealing with each second as it came, there was no feeling of future or past.

(Parratt 2009, 18)

While being in the moment refers to existence in the here and now, it is also an active and responsive process sometimes referred to as 'dwelling' in the changes of time and space (Merleau-Ponty 2002). Jane's in the moment responsiveness to 'each second as it came' demonstrates how subtle this dwelling with change might be. In contrast, Esther's spiritual experience included active responses to the sensations of labour while still being in the moment; she explains:

It was like a dance ... I was very conscious of performing the pattern of the dance. It was almost ... like I looked forward to a contraction to perform this dance. The contractions became part of it, and I was aware of the beauty and the gracefulness of them, and the rhythm ... It was lovely to close my eyes and go right into myself ... this was a very spiritual birth ... it connected me to my mother, and ... to every woman who had ever given birth, right back to primordial days and into the future as well ...

(McDonald 1992, 98)

A woman's responses to her labour pains are both what initiate being in the moment and regulate how deeply nonordinary the spiritual experience is. Gina describes how unintentional, but releasing, her spiritual experience was:

I was aware of going totally inside myself, inside the experience. The rational mind stayed out and I jumped in. I felt like an animal ... I completely let go to a higher power ... it was letting myself be out of control, although it wasn't intentional ... it was a reaction to the pain. I was as deeply inside myself as I needed to be according to the pain that I had; there was no need to go any deeper ... I wasn't focused in my mind, I was down lower, around my heart. It felt so lovely and right.

(Parratt 2009, 209–210)

Being in the moment of spiritual experience is, nonetheless, not one of shutting out the mind to passively succumb to bodily processes. Elizabeth made a choice to focus attention in the present, despite potential distractions within her environment, as she explains:

The contractions felt really intense ... I just stayed in the moment and didn't think too much at all ... I remember ... thinking 'it's all right it only lasts now and it'll change' ... I felt really present and ... also very expansive ... it's like two things happening at once ... I was just aware of my immediate surroundings, I could hear what was going on but I wasn't paying that much attention ... a contraction would come along; I'd grab Bob's hands, stand up with my legs open and 'rahhhh'. Wow, right here!

(Parratt 2009, 54)

In each of these descriptions of being in labour, although the woman is experiencing labour pains she also has a positive sense of connection to herself as an embodied being 'in the moment' of labour. Often there is also a sense of connection to the baby as an entity and a physical connection to the labour partner. Conversely a woman's sense of herself in labour can be compromised by less empowering connections with her environment and the people in that environment.

Feeling safe

A woman's sense of safety, for herself and her baby, is crucial to commencing and then sustaining the focus of being in the moment of a spiritual experience during labour (Parratt and Fahy 2004, Fahy et al. 2011). While only the individual woman can say how safe she feels at any particular time, women are more likely to feel safe and confident if their environment feels like a sanctum: comfortable, familiar and private (Fahy et al. 2011). Within that environment, a woman should also feel holistically safe enough to labour in whatever way that feels right to her. Her feeling of being 'holistically safe' draws from the sensations of her whole embodied self, not merely her ego-centred power that can rationalise away fear or create it. To feel holistically safe, the woman needs to be freed from disempowering interactions where ego-centric powers dominate, and her intrinsic power must be nurtured. Feeling safe enough in labour therefore requires the woman to have jurisdiction over her environment (Fahy et al. 2011).

The midwifery theory 'Birth Territory' further explains that a woman's midwife will ideally act as the guardian of both the physical elements of the birth environment as well as the way power is used in that environment (Fahy et al. 2011). Midwives and other people's use of power within the birth environment can impact on the labouring woman's spiritual experience, her sense of connection and her access to intrinsic power (Parratt 2010). Louise illustrates:

I ... went totally inside myself ... I started imagining where the baby was, I felt like I knew exactly where the top of his head was ... it was ... like a feeling of a big round egg of black energy opening ... it was around the vaginal area and the blackness was spinning slowly and strongly like a downward corkscrew from my left to the right. Then [the midwife] said 'I can see the head' and I was suddenly outside of myself imagining the baby's head coming out; that was the part I'd been scared of. I didn't really feel like I was going through it anymore ... I was an observer looking from the outside ... detached from the whole giving birth experience as well as from the baby.

(Parratt 2009, 78–79)

The comment by Louise's midwife frightens Louise out of a deep and powerful spiritual experience. Louise had not developed a trusting or respectful relationship with her midwife. The midwife was not aware of Louise's fear, so rather than basing the decision to speak on a knowledge of Louise's individual needs, the midwife appears to impose her own interpretation on Louise by assuming she is the same as other women in labour. Although unintentional, in speaking as she did, the midwife used egoic power – that ego-centric power that tends to dominate and consider itself above others; this power communicated disrespect for the uniquely embodied experience of Louise. The impact on Louise was profound; she went into a dissociative state, disconnecting from her intrinsic power and from her baby.

Dissociation is a protective nonordinary conscious state that can be caused by links between past traumatic experiences, such as abuse, and the currently experienced labour; it is a recognised psychological coping strategy in situations where no physical escape is apparent (Parratt 1994, Lanius 2015). Dissociation during labour may also be prompted by the loss in bodily power due to medical intervention, such as an epidural (Akrich and Pasveer 2004). For some women, the protective effect of dissociation means they perceive childbirth positively; however, women who are aware of the link to past trauma, seem to find the experience negative (Parratt 1994). Louise's experience of dissociation shows how women immersed in the moment of spiritual experience are vulnerable to the actions of other people in their environment.

A woman's relationship with her midwife can impact on how labour proceeds. When midwives choose to interact in ways that are empowering, women are more likely to feel holistically safe and capable (Parratt 2010). Midwives need to genuinely explore their own fears and expectations so that their egoic power opens to considering a woman's 'in the moment situation'. During each interaction, midwives will ideally consider both their expert knowledge and the unique aspects of the woman in her individual situation. Decisions made by the midwife are then more likely be done in consultation with the woman and be appropriate to her particular situation; in doing so, midwives will also be able to provide an honest rationale for their actions. Then, the midwife will fully engage with the woman, working mindfully with the woman's power, drawing from and integrating the midwife's own power and/or the power of others such as the partner. Celeste's midwife draws from both self-trust and trust in Celeste's ability:

> As I screamed in pain, [my midwife] would grab my hand, look me in the eye and say 'it's OK love, you're doing really well'. As soon as she did that the pain of the contractions changed and was almost halved … it felt like she was there for me all day.
>
> *(Parratt 2009, 302)*

To feel safe enough being in the moment during labour, women need to establish a sense of trust with their midwife. Trust is crucial and matters. Without such trust a woman may use her egoic power to be defensive or hypervigilant (Parratt and Fahy 2004, Fahy et al. 2011). A trusting relationship will ideally be formed antenatally and continue through labour, yet this is not always feasible in many models of care. However, I contend that it is possible to develop trust with a previously unknown but genuinely caring midwife during labour. For example, Emily developed trust in her midwife whose 'actions and speech' showed that her midwife was 'absolutely nonjudgmental and in touch with what was going on' (Emily in Parratt 2009, 336). Emily's midwife also demonstrated belief in her ability to labour by working with her and being an advocate as well as by doing 'touching little things' like getting cold face washers (336). Emily's midwife demonstrated genuine care for her as a unique individual which in turn reinforced trust and enabled feelings of safety and of empowerment, despite not knowing her prior to labour.

A woman's sense of safety in labour extends not only to the wellbeing of her baby but also to the wellbeing of her partner. Gina, for example, needed to know her partner was safe before her labour would establish. When she started contracting her partner had an asthma attack, Gina explains: 'The asthma attack turned labour off because I had to protect my family right then … with hindsight I realise that to be in labour it was very important for me to feel safe' (Parratt 2009, 205). Helen was not able to trust in the wellbeing of her partner throughout labour. She felt like she 'had to be capable and strong' for the both of them; as soon as she finished a contraction she would 'reaffirm … connection by checking on him' (Parratt 2009, 413). When a woman is continually vigilant during labour she is unlikely to release and attune herself to spiritual experiences. Some women specifically acknowledge the need to know their partners are being effectively supported so they can feel safe enough to be in the moment during labour (McDonald 1992, Parratt 2009, Vernon 2005, 2006).

Partners need to feel safe enough to 'be there' in labour. Attending labour is likely to be a new and unfamiliar activity for a partner; it can prompt feelings of vulnerability and fear of the unknown (Ledenfors and Berterö 2016). Other fears include those for the wellbeing of woman and baby, of fainting, and of having to handle the birth alone (Vernon 2006). Being well prepared and drawing from the support of a chosen friend or trusted midwife can address many of these issues (Johansson, Fenwick and Premberg 2015). Regardless of their gender, all partners require an honest, nonjudgmental and respectful relationship with a midwife; eye contact, engagement, inclusive behaviours, answers to questions and invitations to participate in the woman's caregiving are important (Dahl et al. 2013, Johansson, Fenwick, and Premberg 2015). Emily's midwife showed her partner how to do helpful things, like sacral pressure; she 'nurtured him by affirming him for what he was doing' and when her midwife said to him '"you're doing so well" … it was from the heart' (Parratt 2009, 336–337). When partners feel safe, well supported and prepared they are more able to 'be there', fully present with the labouring woman.

Significance of partners 'being there'

'Being there' with the labouring woman refers to partners' presence physically, emotionally and spiritually, to the very best of their ability. The idea of 'presence' means giving of the self so as to be fully available and responsive to the labouring woman (Pembroke and Pembroke 2008). The experience can be a profound one for the partner both in meeting the baby and in coming to know the labouring woman in a new way (Kainz, Eliasson and von Post 2010, Lahood 2006). Gordon suddenly felt changed 'forever' because of his experience; he explains: 'I experienced this primal condition of fertilising an egg, of becoming a father ... suddenly connected to the whole universe' (Lahood 2006, 18). The change for Dave was in how he perceived his partner; he observes: 'I knew my wife well; however, I had never seen the sort of resilience that she displayed through the birth. She was truly amazing' (Vernon 2006, 129). The partner's experience is also likely to be a challenging one.

When focusing on the labouring woman, partners are challenged to be aware of and negotiate past their own egoic fears and expectations. Steve recognises that his 'dreams' of how labour was 'supposed to be' were 'falling apart'; the process of changing these perceptions was 'like a death really', a spiritual experience 'induced by ... the physical-ness' of his partner giving birth (Lahood 2006, 12, 17). Change necessarily involves death of the old and birth of the new – whether birth of a new way of being, a new sense of self or a new baby (Lacan 1977, Kristeva 1982). As his son is born, Geoffrey realises the link between birth and death; he says it was 'like a shock' as he became aware that 'this child was mortal ... birth is death ... I knew I could not protect him from death' (Lahood 2006, 14–15). Ken also describes a realisation that 'life and death' are 'the same thing' at the moment of birth; however, to him it was an experience of being on 'a knife edge' (Lahood 2006, 9). Ken explains:

> There's a kind of holy instant ... I think of [as] the concept of the past meeting the future, in that moment ... the two meet and then it opens to something else. Like there's another dimension in there ... I suppose that's what people mean by being in the now.
>
> *(Lahood 2006, 9)*

Labours can be long and arduous whether for the woman or her partner; there can be a sense of being 'captured' in labour's intensity (Ledenfors and Berterö 2016, 29, Parratt 2010). Both Andrew and Caroline were immersed, being in the moment of her labour; Andrew explains: 'We got to this flat period ... we'd lost track of time and place ... lost our focus ... it's as though we got so obsessed ... we forgot about the baby' (McDonald 1992, 127). Something needed to change and it came to them in the form of another midwife who brought in 'new energy' reminding them about the baby and empowering Caroline to 'become one with the body again' (127–129).

The physical, emotional and spiritual challenges of labour can not only lower energy levels and prompt feelings of being powerless, they can combine with fear to create a 'crisis of confidence' (Reiger and Dempsey 2006). Jane feared being responsible for pushing her baby out; she resisted the pushing urges and chose to be alone with her partner. She clarifies that her partner 'was really anxious' and 'tried to be supportive but with every contraction [Jane] was saying "I can't do it"' (Parratt 2009, 21). Jane admits she chose him because 'rather than make me face the fear; I knew he would agree with my beliefs that I couldn't do it' (21). Expressions of sympathy, concern or anxiety are unhelpful during a 'crisis of confidence' because they 'reiterate' the labouring woman's perception that she 'can't do it any more' (Reiger and Dempsey 2006, 371). In Jane's situation, her midwives stepped in to share the responsibility and guide them through the pushing phase.

Partners may also have a sense of powerless inadequacy when faced with a labouring woman's pain (Ledenfors and Berterö 2016); it can be a reason why some partners feel reticent about being there at all (Parratt 2009). Rick experiences 'a sense of helplessness, of seeing the woman I love in so much pain and not being able to share this burden' (Vernon 2006, 141). Yet partners can and do effectively 'share the burden' by staying there and being with the labouring woman. Dean explains: 'All you need to do is be there in body and spirit for your beloved. Listen to them. Trust them and help them trust themselves because they can do amazing things' (Vernon 2006, 78).

When a woman is being in the moment of a spiritual experience, the presence of her partner can be profoundly important to her. For Celeste: '[What] helped was Henry's consistency; he didn't leave my side … towards the end I wouldn't let him leave my side, he was part of my security … he was brilliant' (Parratt 2009, 301). A partner can provide security by being a familiar and constant presence who is aware of the woman's wishes and can even advocate for her (Kainz, Eliasson and von Post 2010). Indeed, a partner is likely to have an intimate understanding of the labouring woman which can enhance the couples' verbal and nonverbal communication skills and their responsivity to each other (Bowman, McDonald and Fitzgerald 2015).

Partners can be guided from one moment to the next by the situation of the labouring woman: the sounds she is making, expressions on her face, how she is moving. Rather than comparing her current state with her usual not-in-labour state, the partner can look for subtle differences in movement, tone and expression compared to only a few minutes ago. Where possible a partner will mirror the woman's mode of communication, consider her movements and take care with body language: avoid showing fear but not by being dishonest. While being in the moment Sheila would periodically follow a contraction with a single direction, such as 'change'; her partner Aidan would respond with equally brief alternatives: 'I would say, "shower" or "bedroom"; or "stand up" or "lie down"' (McDonald 1992, 121). Aidan then picked up on what Sheila did or did not want by watching her body language. There were also times where

Sheila said 'I can't do it' but Aidan soon talked her out of it with the answer 'you *are* doing it' (121).

Partners can have a 'special ability' that inspires the labouring woman's 'faith in herself' and empowers her to continue despite feelings of impossibility (Kainz, Eliasson and von Post 2010, 628). Although such an ability might be special it can also be simple; for Debra it just took a whispered message from her husband: '[O]ne more big long push and it's out, you know Deb!' (Vernon 2005, 99). Drawing forth this ability can mean that partners need to learn to manage their own fears first. This is about turning to a special mood in and around childbirth beyond everyday concerns so as not to disturb or cover up the significance of the occasion (Crowther, Smythe and Spence 2014). When partners mindfully acknowledge and explore their fears, they can ensure that fear does not disrupt the labouring woman's power. Sue's partner Ray became quite scared something was wrong when she was 'hooked ... up to a drip' and the baby's heart was monitored. Rather than allowing the fears to take over, Ray quietly gained reassurance from the midwives; he explained: 'I kept these feelings to myself to keep Sue calm' (Vernon 2006, 71).

Sometimes a fear can be countered with logic, Cameron reasoned: 'When you don't really know what to expect, neither do you really know what not to expect' (Vernon 2006, 13). Alternatively, partners might shift a broad, abstract fear such as the sense of responsibility for parenthood toward a specific focus on the current situation. Fears about getting through labour, whether coming from the labouring woman or from her partner, can be alleviated by short phrases used as a personal mantra or as a reminder when necessary. Louise, remembered 'it's only 24 hours of your life' and 'you can bear it', whereas Helen repeated 'this too shall pass' (Parratt 2009, 76, 411). In the final moments of labour, Andrew was challenged by the need to support the whole of his partner Caroline's weight; their baby's birth 'was fantastic' but he said 'the pain ... in my arms was unbelievable' so Andrew maintained the thought 'I've got to stay here' (McDonald 1992, 128).

By finding a way to manage the challenges and fears, partners are more able to bring their whole self to 'being there' during labour. Partners can themselves feel empowered to work with the woman; they can labour together in ways that reflexively inspire and guide each other. Such an endeavour can enable a partner to authentically respond to the uniquely embodied behaviours of the labouring woman, avoiding conformist actions and helping her to create the best possible, individually appropriate environment for birth. Then, during the spiritual experiences at that birth, the new and powerful sense of their own accomplishment is revealed along with the wonder of connection to new life. David's words give further insight:

> I felt ... delight, awe and even ecstasy ... we had created our child and we had birthed our child, our way. What responsibility for the birth we had taken ... it was 'our' baby in all senses of the word. Writing this ... still

brings tears to my eyes. I had a mingling of love … for my baby … for my beautiful wife who had worked so hard … and love for me too. Love that I had been open minded enough to learn … had been brave enough and determined enough to see it through.

(Vernon 2006, 30)

In conclusion, women and partners' spiritual experiences at birth can be profound. These experiences are different from the rationality of ordinary experiences. The contractions of a labouring woman can shift her awareness toward the nonrational focus of being in the moment of a spiritual experience. Nonetheless, there is a vulnerability in being immersed in the depths of spiritual experience so midwives are entrusted with ensuring that the labouring woman feels safe and empowered. A trusting midwife-woman relationship is as important to the woman as the midwife's support of her partner. This chapter has given practical suggestions on how partners, midwives and others can bring their whole self to 'being there' and honouring the sacred nature of birth. By responding to the unfolding moments of labour in the most individually appropriate way for the uniquely embodied woman with whom they are relating, each person present can be touched by the awe-inspiring power of birth and the wonder of new life; in the words of Debra:

With a deep breath, another contraction, a huge long push and a loud roar, my daughter … was born … Fantastic! Unreal! Oh what a feeling! … overwhelming joy and love for everyone in the room coupled with enormous relief, energy and a multitude of other positive emotions.

(Vernon 2005, 99–100)

References

Akrich, M. and Pasveer, B. 2004. 'Embodiment and disembodiment in childbirth narratives.' *Body & Society* 10 (2/3):63–84. doi: 10.1177/1357034X04042935.

Bowman, S., McDonald, S. and Fitzgerald, L. 2015. 'First-time fathers' making a difference during labour and birth.' *Women and Birth* 28, Supplement 1:S8. doi: http://dx.doi.org/10.1016/j.wombi.2015.07.036.

Chen, K. 2004. 'An analytic review of studies on measuring effects of external QI in China.' *Alternative Therapies in Health & Medicine* 10 (4):38–50.

Crowther, S., Smythe, L. and Spence, D. 2014. 'Mood and birth experience.' *Women and Birth* 27 (1):21–25. doi: 10.1016/j.wombi.2013.02.004.

Dahl, B., Fylkesnes, A.M., Sørlie, V. and Malterud, K. 2013. 'Lesbian women's experiences with healthcare providers in the birthing context: A meta-ethnography.' *Midwifery* 29 (6):674–681. doi: 10.1016/j.midw.2012.06.008.

Davis, E. 1989. *Women's intuition.* Berkeley, CA: Celestial Arts.

Dooley, J. 1993. 'Timon's birth story.' *Birth Support Bendigo Newsletter* December (Summer):3–4.

Fahy, K., Parratt, J., Foureur, M. and Hastie, C. 2011. 'Birth territory: A theory for midwifery practice.' In *Theory for midwifery practice*, edited by R. Bryar and M. Sinclair, pp. 215–240. Basingstoke: Palgrave.

Grof, S. 1988. *The adventure of self-discovery*. Albany, NY: State University of New York Press.

Grosz, E. 2004. *The nick of time. Politics, evolution and the untimely*. Crows Nest, NSW: Allen & Unwin.

Harrison, K. and Fahy, K. 2005. 'Feminist and postmodern approaches to qualitative research.' In *Research methods in the sports sciences: Quantitative and qualitative approaches*, edited by G. Tenenbaum and M. Driscoll, pp. 702–738. Aachen, Germany: Meyer and Meyer Sport.

Heron, J. 1992. *Feeling and personhood: Psychology in another key*. Thousand Oaks, CA: Sage Publications.

Irigaray, L. 1993. *An ethics of sexual difference*. Translated by Carolyn Burke and Gillian C. Gill. London: Athlone.

Irigaray, L. 1996. *I love to you: Sketch for a felicity within history*. Translated by Alison Martin. New York: Routledge.

Irigaray, L. 2002. *To speak is never neutral*. Translated by Gail Schwab. New York: Routledge.

Johansson, M., Fenwick, J. and Premberg, Å. 2015. 'A meta-synthesis of fathers' experiences of their partner's labour and the birth of their baby.' *Midwifery* 31 (1):9–18. doi: http://dx.doi.org/10.1016/j.midw.2014.05.005.

Jordan, J. 1991. 'The relational self: A new perspective for understanding women's development.' In *The self: Interdisciplinary approaches*, edited by J. Strauss and G.R. Goethals, pp. 136–149. New York: Springer-Verlag.

Kainz, G., Eliasson, M. and von Post, I. 2010. 'The child's father, an important person for the mother's well-being during the childbirth: A hermeneutic study.' *Health Care for Women International* 31 (7):621–635. doi: 10.1080/07399331003725499.

Kovel, J. 1991. *History and spirit: An inquiry into the philosophy of liberation*. Boston, MA: Beacon Press.

Kristeva, J. 1982. *Powers of horror: An essay on abjection*. New York: Columbia University Press.

Lacan, J. 1977. *Écrits: a selection*. Translated by Alan Sheridan. London: Tavistock Publications.

Lahood, G. 2006. 'Skulls at the banquet: Near birth as nearing death.' *Journal of Transpersonal Psychology* 38 (1). www.atpweb.org/jtparchive/trps-38-01-001.pdf.

Lanius, R.A. 2015. 'Trauma-related dissociation and altered states of consciousness: A call for clinical, treatment, and neuroscience research.' *European Journal of Psychotraumatology* 6 (1): 27905. doi: 10.3402/ejpt.v6.27905.

Ledenfors, A. and Berterö, C. 2016. 'First-time fathers' experiences of normal childbirth.' *Midwifery* 40:26–31. doi: 10.1016/j.midw.2016.05.013.

Leder, D. 1990. *The absent body*. Chicago, IL: University of Chicago Press.

McDonald, V. 1992. *Speaking of birth, an Australian midwife talks with parents about childbirth*. Newham, Victoria: Scribe Publications.

Merleau-Ponty, M. 2002. *The phenomenology of perception*. Translated by Colin Smith. London: Routledge Classics.

Parratt, J. 1994. 'The experience of childbirth for survivors of incest.' *Midwifery* 10 (1):26–39. doi: 10.1016/0266-6138(94)90006-X.

Parratt, J. 2000. 'Trusting enough to be out of control: The impact of childbirth experiences on women's sense of self.' Masters Thesis. Department of Nursing and Midwifery, University of Southern Queensland.

Parratt, J. 2008. 'Territories of the self and spiritual practices during childbirth.' In *Birth territory and midwifery guardianship: Theory for practice, education and research*, edited by K. Fahy, M. Foureur and C. Hastie, pp. 39–54. Edinburgh: Elsevier.

Parratt, J. 2009. *Feelings of change: Stories of having a baby*. Raleigh: Lulu.com.

Parratt, J. 2010. 'Feeling like a genius: Enhancing women's changing embodied self during first childbearing.' PhD Thesis. School of Nursing and Midwifery. The University of Newcastle.

Parratt, J. and Fahy, K. 2004. 'Creating a "safe" place for birth: An empirically grounded theory.' *New Zealand College of Midwives Journal* 30 (1):11–14. Available from www.midwife.org.nz/resources-events/archived-issues.

Parratt, J. and Fahy, K. 2008. 'Including the *non*rational is sensible midwifery.' *Women and Birth* 21 (1):37–42. doi: 10.1016/j.wombi.2007.12.002.

Pembroke, N. and Pembroke, J. 2008. 'The spirituality of presence in midwifery care.' *Midwifery* 24 (3):321–327.

Reiger, K. and Dempsey, R. 2006. 'Performing birth in a culture of fear: An embodied crisis of late modernity.' *Health Sociology Review* 15 (4 Childbirth, Politics & the Culture of Risk):364–373.

Surrey, J. 1991. 'The "self-in-relation": A theory of women's development.' In *Women's growth in connection: Writings from the Stone Center*, edited by J. Jordan, A. Kaplan, J. Baker Miller, I. Stiver and J. Surrey, pp. 51–66. New York: The Guilford Press.

Taylor, K. 1995. *The ethics of caring*. Santa Cruz, CA: Hanford Mead Publishers.

Tzu, L. 1963. *Tao Tê Ching*. Translated by D.C. Lau. London: Penguin Classics.

Vernon, D. ed. 2005. *Having a great birth in Australia*. Canberra, Australia: Australian College of Midwives.

Vernon, D. ed. 2006. *Men at birth*. Canberra, Australia: Australian College of Midwives.

Weedon, C. 1997. *Feminist practice and poststructuralist theory*. 2nd edn. Cambridge, MA: Blackwell.

Wilhelm, R. and Baynes, C. eds. 1967. *The I Ching or Book of Changes*. 3rd edn. *Bollingen Series XIX*. Princeton, NJ: Princeton University Press.

9

SPIRITUAL OBSTETRICS

Alison Barrett

It's not for nothing that there's no such book called *Spiritual Obstetrics*. *Spiritual Midwifery*, on the other hand, is the well-known home birth manual first written by Ina May Gaskin and published in 1975 (Gaskin 1975). Ina May self-trained as a lay midwife to serve the population of hippies to which she belonged. The group travelled across the USA in a convoy of caravans, and eventually settled in an intentional community known today as The Farm. Ina May described the first birth that she ever attended. When one of the women who was travelling with the group unexpectedly went into labour, Ina May's husband Stephen, the spiritual leader of the community, was called to come as no one knew what else they should do. Though Ina May had given birth herself before, in a hospital setting, it is telling that a male authority figure was sought even by this community rather than a woman with personal experience of birth. In any case, when Stephen could not be found Ina May was summoned as a stand in. She describes being transfixed by the experience. She said 'I could not leave even if I wanted to', such was the power of the witnessing.

Ina May's words reveal how birth has the potential power to transform not only women who become mothers in the process, but also the observers who may be either silently traumatised or deeply inspired. Yet as in many potentially transforming experiences, one has to be open to the transformation. The most powerful of experiences can be viewed very differently, and important aspects entirely missed even by people who are present at them. There can be an element of wilful blindness in some cases. As the saying goes, 'there is none so blind as he who will not see'.

Secularisation of birth

The paediatrician Darshak Sanghavi, writing on the pain of childbirth, felt it an evolutionary relic, one that we've risen above with our modern anaesthetics

(Sanghavi 2006). He judged women that embraced the pain of labour and natural childbirth as participants in an extreme and competitive sport. To explain why women would put themselves through this (in his mind) unnecessary pain, he offered the analogy of the festival of Paryushana, an important Janian holy event, where extreme fasting is sometimes practiced (Sanghavi 2006). Extreme fasting, neuroscience tells us, can induce a banquet of neurotransmitter reactions that mimic the ingestion of hallucinogenic substances. Both the substances and the experiences that induce them have been long sought by shamans and medicine men alike. Some would argue that religious seekers and those who experience natural childbirth, are merely inflicting on themselves an idiotic and pointless chemical process. What is suggested by Dr Sanghavi (and he's not the only one with such beliefs), is that both groups of people are duping themselves into accepting as true that experiences of natural childbirth have special meaning (Sanghavi 2006, Talbot 1999). To the nonbeliever, any sort of attempt to become closer to God is merely a fantasy based on a lie. In the case of obstetrics, far from an innocent deception, some in the medical profession feel that the spread of such 'nonsense' might put women and their innocent babies in danger (Kirkup 2015). It is this belief system, ironically an ideology in its own right, that the experience of women should be shelved on an altar of safety and that the empowerment or spiritual growth women experience giving birth under their own terms is a false idol; it is this view that underpins the inherent secularism of obstetrics. It goes some way to explain why there hasn't ever been a book called *Spiritual Obstetrics*.

Nonetheless, spirituality still sneaks in to the birth room, at least occasionally. The French obstetrician Michel Odent noticed the similarities between spontaneous, midwifery attended, uninhibited birth situations, often occurring at home, in comparison to prayer (Odent 2001). He observes in his book *The Scientification of Love* that in such birthing environments women regularly adopt a bending forward position, often kneeling, and that the baby is frequently born as the mother crouches forward (Odent 2001). This contrasts to the preferred positioning of women in a traditional hospital delivery bed, where women are placed on their backs with their feet in stirrups. Odent felt that, in adopting this body stance, people who pray and women who give birth can more easily disassociate from their neocortices, which he believes facilitates the experiences of both (Odent 2001). Birth hormones, Odent and others contend, are largely produced by the more primitive older brain, and are susceptible to inhibition from higher brain functions caused by example from bright lights, conversations, bleeping machinery and fear (Odent 2004, Buckley 2015, Unvas Moberg 2015). Prayer, as in birth, involves silence, stillness and darkness. According to Odent: '[P]raying effectively reduces the activity of the neocortical supercomputer, and may help some people reach another reality, out of space and time' (Odent 2001, 89). By creating the conditions that inhibit prayer, modern obstetric practices maybe be trying to shut out spirituality from the birth room.

Of course, some women bring, or indeed obtain access to, their spiritual selves anyway. They describe birth as being a peak, highly individualised and special experience. They are more than their physiology. Still others realise the only way to have the experience they want and to keep their psyche intact is to birth away from the obstetric gaze, at home. Yet when they do this they risk being shamed.

Birthzillas and birth plans

Obstetric colleges and their chiefs around the world have at times labelled women who chose home birth 'selfish' (O'Leary 2015) for putting their experience ahead of the safety of their baby, (e.g. ACOG 2008) even suggesting that medical opinion should override a woman's human rights (Chervenak et al. 2013). Home birthing women were labelled Birthzillas by the Australian columnist Mia Freedman co-opting the theme of the Bridezilla, a monster-diva who cares more about the (implied trivial) details of her wedding than the significance of the ceremony (Freedman 2012). Interestingly this is exactly the opposite of what many mothers want to accomplish by writing out their birth plans. Rather than merely frivolous event planning, birth plans are tools of hope, akin to written vows, that try to make and hold space for the sacredness of this life event. The default pattern in birthing is anything but sacred. For example, women are exhorted to 'leave their dignity at the door' by many hospital staff as if they and their dignity are two separate individuals, as if they can leave a self that could feel undignified or shamed behind and merely bring their mechanical body to the process of birth. It implies birth in hospital need only involve a body that can be dealt with in a manner that a whole person would find distressing and even un-human.

Unfortunately, in the absence of birth planning, the menu on offer in many hospitals carries with it an implicit agreement to the hospital protocol. Although there is growing multi-disciplinary protocol development it can only be based on available evidence. Sometimes there is very little evidence behind these protocols (Prusova et al. 2014). There remains meagre, poor quality evidence informing policy, some of which can be years out of date. Doctors sometimes do not know the actual data behind the policies they insist on applying for the mother's own good (Olatumbosun, Edouard and Pierson 1998). Labouring women are in no position to ask for references and birth plans provide an opportunity for opting out.

A randomised trial of Taiwanese women showed that women who made birth plans had much more positive birth experiences (there's that word again) than mothers who did not (Kuo et al. 2010). Women who made birth plans reported being grateful for having an open discussion, feeling heard and validated and they felt such plans gave them a chance to air their fears and give the reasons for particular choices. But perhaps Mia Freedman cannot be blamed for her views. In an open editorial in the *Contemporary Ob/Gyn* journal that referenced this research, called 'Don't fear the patient with a birth plan', Dr Yalda Afshar wrote that birth plans are associated with unspoken negativity in delivery staff illustrating a clear disconnect between many obstetricians and their patients (Afshar 2016).

Where does this disconnect come from? It comes from a view that denies women their plans and dreams for their birth as it denies that they have choices. It comes from the belief that having a baby is a mechanical event, a physiological process to be managed using evidence, not a psychological or spiritual one that should be protected in a sacred space and allowed to unfold as it should. It comes from a view of the body as nothing more than a machine, and an unreliable and dangerous one at that. It comes from a place of paternalism: that the only reasonable choice is the one a doctor makes, and women who are reasonable should align their expectations with those choices. It comes from a fear that doctors have of being found out, that is to say – the evidence they hold dear is not as clear as advertised. It comes from the opposite of a spiritual view of obstetrics; it emerges from vigorous attempts at its secularisation.

Organics and mechanics

The late British birth guru and childbirth educator Sheila Kitzinger wrote extensively about women's experiences of birth. During her last Australasian tour in 2007, Sheila was interviewed by prominent New Zealand journalist Carol Hirschfield (Kitzinger 2007). The TV interview had a predictably provocative slant asking whether New Zealand women have become 'too posh to push'. While Sheila spoke of birth as the opportunity to be 'at one with the world and the wind and the mountains and the tides', Carol asked whether women aren't 'more empowered by having more options for the management of birth, options like caesarean section for example'. Obviously the women were speaking two different languages.

These two different languages have been allocated space into the lexicons of native tongues of two different, opposing groups of maternity providers. In 2005, the journalist and author Mary Rose MacColl was commissioned to write a review of the maternity system in Queensland (Cherrell Hirst 2005). During this review, she coined the phrases 'organic' and 'mechanic' to describe what she felt were the two archetypes of birth workers she encountered within the Queensland maternity system. According to MacColl, the mechanics, mainly obstetricians, believe that birth needs to take place surrounded by technology. They believe that (their) expertise can mitigate the unforeseeable risks of pregnancy and birth. The organics, mostly midwives, see birth as a normal life event that should be allowed to unfold on its own. Consequently most midwives believe that birth and pregnancy don't sit well inside the medical model (MacColl 2009).

In some ways, MacColl's stereotyped polarised birthing philosophies delineate the two types of people there are in the world: optimists versus pessimists, spiritualists versus secularists, or believers versus atheists. The mechanics see themselves as 'evidence based' practitioners, having the upper hand of science, and deriding the organics view of the importance of the softer spiritual and experiential aspects of birth as so much 'woo'.

MacColl later expanded this theme in a book called *Birth Wars* (MacColl 2009). Women, she writes, are caught in the crossfire between these two groups, and sometimes they and their babies become a sort of collateral damage. She admits that it's the mechanics who have the upper hand. 'Whatever choices, once they enter the hospital system, what happens to them is prescribed by hospital protocols or an individual obstetrician's preferences' (MacColl 2009, 12). In other words, the mechanics are in charge. MacColl notes that something important is lost in this system when she remarks that though 'nowadays in some hospitals there are prints on softly painted walls and husbands in the delivery rooms, but this pays little more than lip service to the notion that childbirth is a key life experience for women and families' (MacColl 2009).

Safety and choice

The issue of the importance of the transformational and spiritual aspects of women's birth experiences is all too often dismissed on the grounds of safety. Take the often repeated phrase 'a healthy baby is all that matters', which sums up a common view that women should give up the idea that birth should be or in fact can be, so much more than the extraction of a live baby from their bodies. Milli Hill writes that 'Taken to the extreme, this idea that the woman does not matter as long as the baby is healthy can create an environment in which her autonomy over her own body is completely lost' (Hill 2015). If there is even a very small risk to the baby, what is justifiable? While some women don't want or seek a spiritual birthing experience, others do. When such experiences are denied, trauma can result. Hill writes,

> [I]f we continue to repeat that a healthy baby is all that matters, we open the doors for all manner of undignified or even abusive treatment to happen to women in the quest for absolute safety. We reduce a woman to being a mere 'vessel' for her child, and we quickly silence anyone who wishes to protest against any aspect of their care that they didn't feel comfortable with.
>
> *(Blog: Milli Hill 2015)*

This is because we can always pull out the dead baby card to shame them. Doctors often overblow the risk of harm in birth in order to frighten women into compliance with hospital protocols, and shame them into giving up their selfish wishes for a personalised experience, something Odent has called 'obstetric scare'. In spite of the fact that much of the evidence on which these protocols are based is often of very poor quality (Wright et al. 2011, Foureur et al. 2010, Prusova et al. 2014). Yet even if the evidence for such harm was robust, the woman should still get to decide.

Challenges of being a spiritual obstetrician

As Karen Armstrong, author of *Twelve Steps to a Compassionate Life*, wrote, 'If it is not tempered by compassion and empathy, reason can lead men and women into a moral void (Armstrong 2011, 86). The moral void, if it had a shape, might take the form of an obstetrician. Yet, this does not apply to all obstetricians. As they say on social media #notallobstetricians. Michel Odent says, 'A human being cannot be a "person" all the time. It would be exhausting'. He points out that the word person comes from the Latin 'persona', a mask adopted by actors (Odent 2001, 80). If obstetricians are at all times to be persons, in other words, to deny their spiritual selves, to place on their faces a mask of evidence base – do they become exhausted? It is interesting to note that burnout in the obstetric profession is rife (Peckham 2013).

Robin Youngson, the founder of Hearts in Health care, summarised the problem with the way medicine is currently practiced during a recent interview with Dr Paddy Barrett on The Doctor Paradox (Youngson 2016). Youngson pointed out that that the origins of the current problems in medicine started in the last century, when a technological model was adopted. The view of the body as a machine held the promise that we might discover all of its secrets and therefore, be able to fix any of its problems. Things came completely undone when we believed that technology would solve everything. Medicine became disease focused instead of health focused (Youngson 2016). All the while we doctors have focused on the wrong things, in treating diseases instead of treating human beings.

Meanwhile, the experiences of women continue to be denied. When research came out which confirmed that some women have orgasms during childbirth (Postel 2013), many internet doctor groups dismissed the idea as ridiculous. It reminded me of the Steve Martin joke: 'You know that look that a woman gets in her eyes when she wants to have sex? Me neither.' Doctors who can't contemplate orgasmic birth remain incredulous about it because it's not in the realm of possibility in their own experience.

I remember joining a group of women who were in the midst of a conversation about being with women at birth. They were talking about the sexual things they'd seen in the birth room, feeling at times voyeurs. They spoke of seeing women moaning, swaying and closing their eyes. I had been at these births too. Called to quietly review a foetal heart tracing, the midwife and I would exchange a knowing look: this birth is going to go fine. But as the conversation about such sightings in birthing rooms went on, an obstetrician in the group grew quiet and left quickly.

I was later told that doctor had just shared her own birth story with the group. She had experienced most of the cascade … induction, and then, all the usual embellishments, IV oxytocin, meconium, foetal heart rate decelerations, scalp electrode, episiotomy, forceps … 'Why anyone would even *want* natural childbirth, and put their child's life at risk, is just beyond me,' she had just been saying.

I have no doubt that some doctors never come to know that there could be so much more to birth than the production of a healthy child. These colleagues never see the sacred power of women in the birth rooms when they enter, therefore they simply do not believe it exists. Crowther, Smythe and Spence (2014) found that those who are at birth, including obstetricians, need to turn to and attune to birth's specialness lest the sacred mood or quality be left hidden, lost, covered over and ignored. I saw one unbeliever, with an entourage of students surrounding her, march into a birth room where the midwife had tried to carefully hold the woman's space, and declare 'There'll be none of that nonsense here'. There must be a protective effect in convincing oneself, as one goes about performing interventions that harm, that a healthy baby is all that matters. But what happens when you are made aware of what you have lost?

Personally, I feel sorry for the mechanics – among them, many fellow obstetricians. As the poet and philosopher Criss Jami said: 'When good people consider you the bad guy, you develop the heart to help the bad ones' (Jami 2015, 92). I am an obstetrician, I belong to the college; I'm one of their fellowship, a member of their body.

I look to Sara Miles (Miles 2007), the left-leaning lesbian Christian activist and writer. She says that people ask her how someone like her can belong to a group like them. By which she means the group of right wing, bigoted, mean and nasty hypocrites who call themselves followers of Jesus. She explains that an essential part of being a Christian is having to embrace the other Christians. You don't get to pick and choose. In her definition of Christianity, you have to love everyone when you sign up for it (Miles 2007). Those fellow deplorables are your kin, sinners all.

There is no such rule in obstetric colleges. But there is a similar form of excommunication that can occur when you don't subscribe to all the views held by your peers. And yet, the overlying scripture we are supposed to be following is at the very least, about doing no harm and at most, advocating for the best possible outcomes for mothers and their babies. In both the Church of Obstetricians and the Church of God, it comes down to how you interpret the literature. At that same conference, I was asked why many of my fellow obstetricians do not see the same things I see. I figure it is because they apply love exactly the wrong way, just like the bad Christians do.

I leave you with a birth story. Some say every birth is an ordinary miracle. Others say birth is an ordinary life event. This birth was neither miraculous nor ordinary, and it was certainly one that I will never forget.

My midwife friend Karen had this patient she was really nervous about. It was her second baby and everything was going well. But when this woman booked in for care she told Karen that back when she was 8 years old, she'd gone to see a fortune teller. This fortune teller had told her that her second baby would die during childbirth. What kind of fortune teller tells an 8 year old that her future baby is going to die? I mean, are there no codes of ethics for fortune tellers?

In the New Zealand maternity system, there are strict guidelines for midwifery referrals to obstetricians. These guidelines cover blood pressure problems, growth problems, a long list of indicators of maternal and foetal well-being. There is nothing on the list about the premonitions of fortune tellers. I told Karen, 'You might order an extra a scan or two. Just to make sure the growth is okay.' And it was.

I forgot about all of this. One day I was leaving work through the back door of the hospital, and my friend Karen was coming in with a woman. The woman was bent over, with a blood soaked towel between her legs. Karen said, 'Don't go.' I followed them down the hall into the caesarean section theatre. Someone rang the emergency bell. Someone else tried to find the baby's heartbeat. Many people came, but time was being wasted. I heard myself saying, 'She's not quite fully, but I think I can pull the baby out.' With one pull, the baby came. Pale and lifeless, the paediatricians began resuscitation.

But the woman said, 'It's dead isn't it? I know it's dead. The fortune teller told me so.'

It was then that I realised that this was that woman, the same woman Karen had told me about.

Later, we looked at the placenta. A tiny blood vessel, carrying foetal blood, ran in the membranes around the baby, and when the waters broke, this little blood vessel ruptured and the baby exsanguinated. There was nothing to be done; it was a random event, the kind of thing that was as rare and likely as being struck by lightning. When I told the woman this, by way of a clumsy attempt at comfort, she told me that she had once been struck by lightning too.

References

ACOG . 2008. 'ACOG statement on home births.' ACOG News Release. Washington, 6 February.

Afshar, Y. 2016. 'Don't fear the patient with a birth plan.' *Contemporary Ob/Gyn*. http://contemporaryobgyn.modernmedicine.com/contemporary-obgyn/news/don-t-fear-patient-birth-plan.

Armstrong, K. 2011. *Twelve Steps to a Compassionate Life*. London: Random House.

Buckley, S.J. 2015. *Hormonal physiology of childbearing: Evidence and implications for women, babies, and maternity care*. Washington, DC: Childbirth Connections. http://www.nationalpartnership.org/research-library/maternal-health/hormonal-physiology-of-childbearing.pdf.

Cherrell Hirst, A.O. 2005. Re-birthing report of the review of maternity services in Queensland. Government review, Queensland Government.

Chervenak, F.A., McCollough, L.B., Brent, R.L., Levene, M.I. and Arabin, B. 2013. 'Planned home birth: The professional responsibility response.' *American Journal of Obstetrics & Gynecology* 208 (1): 31–38. doi: 10.1016/j.ajog.2012.10.002.

Crowther, S., Smythe, L. and Spence, D. 2014. 'Mood and birth experience.' *Women and Birth: Journal of the Australian College of Midwives* 27 (1): 21–25.

Foureur, M., Ryan, C., Nicholl, M. and Homer, C. 2010. 'Inconsistent evidence: Analysis of six national guidelines for vaginal birth after cesarean section.' *Birth* 37 (1): 3–10. doi: 10.1111/j.1523-536X.2009.00372.x.

Freedman, M. 2012. 'Birthzillas: When it's all about the birth, not the baby.' Mamamia! What women are talking about. 18 June. Accessed 8 August 2016. www.mamamia.com. au/birthzillas-its-about-the-birth-not-the-baby/.

Gaskin, I.M. 1975. *Spiritual Midwifery*. Summertown, TN: Book Publishing Company.

Hill, M. 2015. The positive birth movement. 12 December. Accessed 8 August 2016. www. positivebirthmovement.org/pbm-blog.

Jami, C. 2015. *Killosophy*. CreateSpace Independent Publishing Platform.

Kirkup, B. 2015. *The report of the Morecambe Bay investigation.* London: The Stationery Office.

Kitzinger, S. Interview by Carol Hirschfeld. Campbell Live (3 November 2007).

Kuo, S.C., Lin, K.C., Hsu, C.H., Yang, C.C., Chang, M.Y., Tsao, C.M. and Lin, L.C. 2010. 'Evaluation of the effects of a birth plan on Taiwanese women's childbirth experiences, control and expectations fulfilment: a randomised controlled trial.' *International Journal of Nursing Studies* 47 (7): 806–814. doi: 10.1016/j.ijnurstu.2009.11.012.

MacColl, M.R. 2009. *The birth wars*. St. Lucia: The University of Queensland Press.

Miles, S. 2007. *Take this bread*. New York: Ballantine Books.

Odent, M. 2001. *The scientification of love*. London: Free Association Books.

Odent, M. 2004. *The caesarean*. Sidmouth: Free Association Books.

Olatunbosun, O.A., Edouard, L. and Pierson, R.A. 1998. 'Physicians' attitudes toward evidence based obstetric practice: a questionnaire survey.' *British Medical Journal* (January 31), 316 (7128): 365–366.

O'Leary, C. 2015. 'Homebirths a "selfish" risk.' 7 July. Accessed 8 August 2016. https:// au.news.yahoo.com/thewest/wa/a/28685846/homebirth-a-selfish-risk/#page1.

Peckham, C. 2013. 'Ob/Gyn lifestyles – linking to burnout: A Medscape survey.' Medscape. 28 March. Accessed 8 August 2016. www.medscape.com/features/slideshow/ lifestyle/2013/womens-health.

Postel, T. 2013. 'Childbirth climax: The revealing of obstetrical orgasm.' *Sexologies* 22 (4): e89–e92.

Prusova, K., Churcher, L., Tyler, A. and Lokugamage, A.U. 2014. 'Royal College of Obstetricians and Gynaecologists guidelines: How evidence-based are they.' *Journal of Obstetrics and Gynecology* 34 (8): 706–711.

Sanghavi, D. 2006. 'The motherlode of pain.' *Boston Globe*, 23 July.

Talbot, M. 1999. 'The way we live now: Pay on delivery.' *New York Times Magazine*, 1999 October.

Unvas Moberg, K. 2015. 'How kindness, warmth, empathy and support promote the progress of labor.' In *The roar behind the silence: How kindness, compassion and respect matter in maternity*, by Sheena Byrom and Soo Downe, p. 250. London: Pinter & Martin.

Wright, J.D., Pawar, N., Gonzalez, J.S., Lewin, S.N., Burke, W.M., Simpson, L.L., Charles, A.S., D'Alton, E.E. and Hertzog T.J. 2011. 'Scientific evidence underlying the American College of Obstetricians and Gynecologists' practice bulletins.' *Obstetrics and Gynecology* 118 (3): 505–512.

Youngson, R. 2016. Interview by Paddy Barrett. Rehumanizing Healthcare (11 September).

10

GROWTH AND RENEWAL THROUGH TRAUMATIC BIRTH

Gill Thomson

In the literature, a 'normal' (i.e. vaginal, intervention-free) childbirth event is heralded as the gold standard; a birth imbued with personal and spiritual growth and positive adaption to the parenting role (Mauger 2000). A medicalised/interventionist birth on the other hand is associated with a loss of spirituality and psychological adversity. However, in my and others' research, there are stories that reveal how all types of birth ('normal' or otherwise) can be experienced as negative/traumatic events, and how these births can create new purpose and meaning. Complex and complicated births are often construed as growth-restricting due to a false dichotomous understanding of spiritual as something only connected to 'normal' births. In this chapter I offer a different perspective by illuminating how a traumatic birth (normal or otherwise) can create new meanings, possibilities and relationships.

The knowledge that adversity can lead to growth and renewal is archaic. Stressful, difficult events, such as childbirth, can lead to symptoms of post-traumatic stress and/or a clinical diagnosis of post-traumatic stress disorder (PTSD). However, such events also offer the premise for new possibilities and meanings, through post-traumatic growth (PTG). PTG is defined as the 'positive psychological change experienced as a result of the struggle with highly challenging life circumstances' (Tedeschi and Calhoun 2004, 1). PTS infers the negative psychosocial implications of a difficult, stressful life event, whereas PTG is how our internal conflicts in the aftermath of trauma can lead to fundamental and transformative alterations in how we perceive ourselves, others, and our life-world.

In the following sections, I highlight why PTG is an important area of study through considering how the current rhetoric falsely dichotomises what constitutes a 'good' birth, as well as how a more salutogenic approach (i.e. one that focuses on factors promoting positive health and wellbeing) (Antonovsky 1979) is required to counteract the pathological focus in perinatal care – an approach that perpetuates fear and risk. I define what PTG is, and outline the current evidence basis of growth within the perinatal area. The five domains of PTG are then used as a theoretical lens to present narrative insights to illuminate how mothers were able to achieve new insights and meanings following a self-defined traumatic birth. I provide a short summary to consider how these insights resonate with the wider spirituality literature. Finally, implications for practice and research in this area are offered.

Why is it important to consider PTG?

In the wider literature a number of authors have considered the spiritual and transcendental nature of childbirth (e.g. Ina May Gaskin, Benig Mauger, Jenny Hall, Lynn Callister, Ruth Tanyi and Trudelle Thomas). These authors highlight how childbirth is an emotional, physical, cognitive and potentially spiritual experience that transcends the physical realms and empowers women. However, it appears that many of these accounts are limited to natural physiological birth. Medicalised births on the other hand are mainly associated with loss of spirituality (Gaskin 1990, Mauger 2000). The rites and rituals of obstetric practice are believed to deplete the spiritual surges during birth, which can leave women feeling alienated and vulnerable (Mauger 2000, Tanyi 2002). Much of the literature thereby upholds a normal vaginal birth as the outcome to aim for, whereas intervention based/medicalised births are believed to pre-dispose psychological morbidity and potential for spiritual distress.

The dualistic conceptions of medicalised/interventionist (bad) and normal physiological (good) binaries of birth are problematic for a number of reasons. First, they offer a limited and restricted focus of modern childbirth which are not reflective of women's diverse birth experiences; women experiencing caesarean sections, instrumental deliveries as well as uncomplicated vaginal births have all reported negative, traumatic experiences (Thomson and Downe 2008, 2010, Beck and Watson 2016). Second, they overlook the potentially positive and rewarding experiences of a medicalised birth for some women (Davis-Floyd 1992, Zadorozynj 1999, Thomson and Downe 2010, Crowther, Smythe and Spence 2014). A further concern is how women can be castigated (by self or others) as victims and failures should interventions, medication and/or personal difficulty form part of their birth experience (Zadorozynj 1999, Frost et al. 2006). This leaves women like Ruth feeling disempowered:

> I felt I had no right to feel like I had because I'd had a normal delivery, nothing bad happened to me, so it felt I wasn't allowed to have such a strong response.
>
> *(Thomson 2007, 239)*

A further caveat in existing maternity care literature is its predominant focus on pathology and adversity (Downe and McCourt 2004). For example, predictors and implications of a traumatic birth/PTSD onset following childbirth (e.g. Ayers et al. 2016, Fenech and Thomson 2014) and fear of birth (FOB) (e.g. Stoll et al. 2014, Ryding et al. 2015) are growing areas of concern. While these areas of research are important for fiscal and moral reasons, it can also be argued how a dominant pathological perspective is perpetuating and magnifying a fear culture.

In this chapter I offer a different perspective. Through drawing on my own PhD study and other available, albeit limited, research, I describe and explore how PTG is experienced by mothers who had a traumatic/distressing birth ('normal' or otherwise). These insights transcend dualistic accounts of childbirth; demonstrate how positive psychological and spiritual growth is not unique to a normal, natural delivery, and offer a more salutogenic perspective of the 'ordinary miracle' (Peterson 1996) of childbirth.

Post-traumatic growth (PTG)

What is PTG? The most recent clinical definition of a traumatic event is one in which the individual has directly or indirectly been exposed to actual or threatened death, serious injury or sexual violation, and which has caused significant distress and impaired functioning (DSM-V; American Psychiatric Association 2013). While trauma obviously creates deep distress and adverse implications for self and others, it also holds transformative powers for positive change through PTG (Tedeschi and Calhoun 2004). The increased interest in PTG forms part of the 'positive psychology' movement (Tedeschi and Calhoun 2004) or what Antonovksy (1979) refers to as a salutogenic orientation. Antonovsky's (1979) seminal work with holocaust survivors led him to postulate that while stressors are omnipresent in our life-worlds, it is how we perceive, internalise and 'cope' with these events that determines our physical and mental outcomes.

A similar related concept relates to resilience, 'the ability of an individual to respond positively and consistently to adversity, using effective coping strategies' (Hunter and Warren 2014, 927). Being 'resilient' means that we have the psychological strength to respond to and cope with stressful and negative life events. In a childbirth-related context, high levels of resilience have been significantly associated with reduced depression levels and higher mental quality of life (Mautner et al. 2013). A resilience-informed PTSD intervention framework was also found to be effective, albeit among those who had no previous mental illness (Turkstra et al. 2013).

PTG, however, offers something more ontologically meaningful. Coping and resilience are considered to hold restorative functions in terms of individuals having the internal and external resources to effectively respond to stressful situations in order to retain their previous level of functioning (Tedeschi and Calhoun 2004). PTG on the other hand goes beyond restoring the 'disequilibrium caused by the traumatic event' (Black and Sandelowski 2010, 228); rather it is a transformative transcendent experience with salutary implications for new growth potential (Tedeschi and Calhoun 2004). While PTG is not considered

TABLE 10.1 Post-traumatic growth inventory (Tedeschi and Calhoun 1996)

Domain	Overview
Relating to others (7 items)	Development of more meaningful and reciprocal relationships
Personal strength (4 items)	Increased self-reliance, acceptance and personal strength to overcome challenges
Spiritual change/development (2 items)	A stronger faith and understanding of spiritual issues
New possibilities (5 items)	New interests and opportunities
Appreciation of life (3 items)	Increased appreciation of what is important in life

to be a universal phenomenon (Tedeschi and Calhoun 1995, Tedeschi, Park and Calhoun 1998), it is purported to occur more distinctively after a severe life crisis (Tedeschi, Calhoun and Groleau 2015).

Tedeschi and Calhoun (1995) identified three broad domains of PTG: relational – more positive, intimate relationships with others; renewed self-perceptions – such as increased self-esteem and sense of personal strength; and alterations to the individual's philosophy of life – such as changes in goals, meaningfulness, expectations and priorities. These areas were used to develop the Post-traumatic Growth Inventory (PTGI; Tedeschi and Calhoun 1996), a 21-item scale which measures growth in five areas (refer to Table 10.1).

Processes underpinning PTG

Tedeschi and colleagues draw on the work of Janoff-Bulman (1992) to outline the processes underpinning PTG. Janoff-Bulman postulates that we hold beliefs and assumptions about ourselves and the world – that we have self-worth, will not experience misfortune and that our life-worlds are 'meaningful' and 'benevolent'. Trauma creates a breach in these assumptions leading to fundamental alterations in our self-perceptions and perceptions of others:

> Traumatic events are atypical in that psychologically we are unprepared for them, they are unrepresented in our assumptive world.
>
> *(Janoff-Bulman 1992, 53)*

Calhoun and Tedeschi (1998) use an earthquake metaphor to emphasise how the traumatic event represents a 'seismic' occurrence that fundamentally alters our life-worlds – an event that leads us to question our purpose, relationships and expectations. This is reflected by Jules, a woman following a traumatic birth:

I can feel just talking about it if I imagine myself 8 months pregnant and feeling and how I was, how I looked, how together I felt and then imagine myself well for months after I didn't recognise myself. Can remember feeling that it had ruined my life, and it was so extreme the change as well. So yeah it feels like a happy together person [...] totally disappeared, I don't know where I went to but I totally disappeared.

(Thomson 2007, 222)

Jules's story depicts a woman who appears broken, in need of rebuilding. 'Rebuilding' (i.e. cognitively and emotionally) subsequently takes place as our schemas and assumptions are revised and reformed (Calhoun and Tedeschi 1998).

Tedeschi and Calhoun (2004) argue that it is how we adopt and respond in the aftermath of a traumatic event, rather than the event itself, that enables growth to occur. PTG is both a process (how growth occurs through an iterative re-evaluation process) and an outcome (fundamental changes to our perspectives, goals and outlooks) (Tedeschi et al. 2015). Growth and distress are also reported to co-exist; with suffering a necessary pre-requisite for growth to occur (Shakespeare-Finch and Lurie-Beck 2014, Tedeschi et al. 2015). For example, we may continue to experience adversity when trying to make sense of the traumatic event, while at the same time it has enabled us to develop new perspectives and beliefs. We may live a deeper and more meaningful existence after a life-shattering event, but it does not necessarily mean that our emotional distress has lessened (Tedeschi et al. 2015).

Post-traumatic growth in the perinatal period

While PTG has been explored following a variety of traumatic life events, such as war, abuse, divorce and bereavement (refer to Tedeschi et al. 2015), to date published reports into PTG following a traumatic birth remain limited. Three quantitative based studies have examined perinatal PTG in community samples of mothers using the PTGI (Sawyer and Ayers 2009, Sawyer et al. 2012, Sawyer et al. 2015). Two of these studies are of particular relevance (Sawyer and Ayers 2009, Sawyer et al. 2012). These UK-based studies identified moderate levels of growth following childbirth (48–50%) and the most endorsed PTG domains were 'appreciation of life' and 'personal strength'. The study by Sawyer and Ayers (2009) also reported similar rates of personal growth between women who did or did not meet PTSD diagnostic criteria (whatever type of birth she experienced). This finding thereby highlights how growth can occur irrespective of women's birth appraisal. PTG in relation to other perinatal areas, such as several fetal diagnosis and perinatal loss are also reported (e.g. Black and Sandelowski 2010, Black and Wright 2012); however, as these experiences are arguably distinct from women who had a self-defined traumatic birth and often achieve optimum outcomes (i.e. a healthy baby), they have not been considered in-depth here.

How women experience PTG following a traumatic birth

In order to appreciate the growth experienced by women following a traumatic birth, it is pertinent to offer some context into how such events are experienced and internalised. A traumatic birth is one imbued with loss of control, isolation, uninformed procedures and poor/negative relationships with care providers; an abusive, devastating, disembodying experience which can lead women to feel totally divorced from the experience of birth (Elmir et al. 2010). Clare, a woman who had had a straightforward vaginal birth illustrates this:

> Don't feel I gave birth and had a baby on that day, I just felt I went into a room and was just assaulted.
>
> *(Clare – Thomson and Downe 2008, 270)*

A meta-synthesis of qualitative studies to explore the psychosocial implications of a traumatic birth, such as Clare's description, reports how these events are associated with anger and self-blame, reduced confidence and self-esteem, social isolation, fractured relationships with infants and partners, classic PTSD symptoms such as violent flashbacks and nightmares, and loss of family ideas as many women chose not to have further children (Fenech and Thomson 2014). It is clear that relationships, connectedness, purpose and meaning can be disrupted in all types of birthing experiences, yet (as discussed later) such changes can lead to the potential for personal growth and renewal.

In this section, I largely draw on my PhD research (Thomson 2007, Thomson and Downe 2010, 2013), and research undertaken by Beck and Watson (2010, 2016). These studies involve women who had a subsequent birth following a self-defined traumatic birth event (Thomson 2007, Thomson and Downe 2010, 2013, Beck and Watson 2010). The women (n = 15) in Beck and Watson's (2016) study were asked to write narratives that detailed any positive changes as a result of their traumatic birth. The women included in these studies had either had a medicalised birth (i.e. caesarean, forceps delivery) or 'normal' vaginal delivery; a few of which were associated with maternal and/or infant morbidities (e.g. postpartum haemorrhage, neonatal unit admission).

In line with the wider PTG literature, the co-existence of distress and renewal was evident in the women's narratives; however, it is the positive elements of growth that I have focused on. The approach adopted by Black and Sandelowski (2010) has been utilised to present case study material within the five PTGI domains (see Table 10.1) to illuminate the transformation, new possibilities and strength that women attained following a self-defined traumatic birth (both following birth trauma and during a future conception).

Appreciation of life

Appreciation of life concerns how we re-evaluate and set new priorities based on what is important in our lives. One of the ways this element of growth was evident in women's accounts was through the notion of fortitude; as Kathy highlights, despite enduring a traumatic, distressing experience, she had been 'lucky' to have a healthy infant:

> You put it in a box [negative emotions], shut the lid, you put it away and think I've got a perfectly healthy baby now, there are people out there who don't have perfectly healthy [babies], I'm the lucky one.
>
> *(Thomson 2007, 237)*

Kathy feeling lucky may not necessarily be unique for women who have experienced a traumatic birth; arguably all birthing women want a healthy baby. However, following trauma, the notion of 'luck', as reported here by Kathy, often represented an important mechanism to re-frame and transcend what women had endured into feeling '*blessed*' for achieving an optimum outcome. Some mothers, like Jules, portray a rather selfless maternal predisposition that accepts sufferance for the ones they love:

> I can remember feeling thank god he's alive thank god he's alright and I'd rather it was me that was in bits than my baby.
>
> *(Thomson 2007, 238)*

There was also evidence of how trauma had enabled women to hold a more appreciative world perspective; to value what they had and to worry about events as they occur. Clare tells us how she came to savour each moment:

> You've just got to make the most of every moment, and not let things worry you and what will be will be, and just take each day as it comes and just enjoy your children. Stop worrying about things, things will be OK as long as you've got the love there and you're together, your own family, then nothing else in the world really matters.
>
> *(Thomson 2007, 298)*

Spiritual change/development

This domain relates to having a greater belief and understanding of spiritual matters. While spirituality is not necessarily associated with religious beliefs and convictions (Greenstreet 2006) some women such as Kate referred to how her faith had helped her 'to get through it [traumatic birth]' (Thomson 2007, 224). One of the mothers in the study by Beck and Watson (2016) also described how her connection to God had become stronger:

> I used to feel that my traumatic birth was something I wanted to take back (to somehow reverse time and change it so I could be 'ME' again) but over time I have learnt to embrace it as it keeps me connected to God and has also been one of the biggest catalysts for positive change in my life.
>
> *(Beck and Watson 2016, 269)*

Other women, such as reflected in the following quote, spoke of how their relationship with God had improved; how their personal deity had enabled them to access the help that they needed, and how their traumatic birth experience and associated spiritual beliefs had provided them with new life directions:

> [B]ut He has also given me huge insight into birth trauma which I hope to use for His glory in helping others with similar experiences.
>
> *(Beck and Watson 2016, 269)*

Personal strength

Personal strength relates to our capacity to deal with and respond to adversities, and an increased sense of self-reliance. This domain was a key area to emerge within the qualitative accounts. Diane for example, described her personal resolve to 'not allow' the emotional dysphoria of her traumatic birth to impact on her maternal experience, or the relationship with her infant:

> I get on with it and cope with it because that's what I have to do and it was very much that with X's [daughter] birth, there was nobody gonna take any of this enjoyment away from me, I'd waited 6 and a half years for her and she's here now she's absolutely gorgeous and I'm not gonna let anything spoil that as far as I can, I'm not gonna let anything spoil that.
>
> *(Diane – Thomson 2007, 240)*

The magnitude of positive growth attained through a traumatic birth is reflected in a quote from one of the mother's in Beck and Watson's study; 'I was broken and now I am unbreakable' (2016, 268). A further woman from this study described how her inner strength had developed through knowing she was able to survive future adversities:

> No one would wish trauma or subsequent PTSD upon anyone, yet when having had this, one knows you have become CHANGED FOREVER yet a better person for it all. Better and stronger and very self-aware undergirds your new daily life.
>
> *(Beck and Watson 2016, 268)*

This inner strength was also evident among women who were preparing for a subsequent birth following a traumatic ordeal. Some spoke of how this represented a 'fight' and a 'battle' to obtain the care and support they needed (Thomson 2007). Jules speaks of a battle that required self-reliance and perseverance:

> You've really got to fight the battle on your own. There is something inside you that you either fight it or go under really.
>
> *(Thomson 2007, 356)*

Women, having similar experiences to Jules, referred to their personal strength in confronting their former adversity; 'to face your fears', even with the knowledge of how harmful a further potentially traumatic event could be to their self-hood; Jules describes this:

> I can remember that was the risk I took having X [daughter – second child], having another baby the risk was that I would disappear and this time I wouldn't come back you know and that … was real to me.
>
> *(Thomson 2007, 359)*

Women's assertiveness developed following a traumatic birth as they learnt to use 'their voice and personal power to fight back emotionally and physically for themselves and others' (Beck and Watson 2016, 268). In my research women used phrases such as 'highly motivated', 'vociferous' and 'determined' to achieve a more positive birth experience (Thomson 2007, 356). A mother in Beck and Watson's (2010) study also reported how she was 'planning for this birth literally while they were stitching me up from the traumatic first birth' (Beck and Watson 2010, 245).

Numerous strategies were employed to achieve a 'different' birth following an occasion of trauma, including: a review of their birth with maternity professionals; visit to the delivery suite; attending further antenatal educational classes; reading texts on birth physiology; creating multiple birth plans for different birth trajectories; and homeopathic-type remedies (Thomson and Downe 2010, Beck and Watson 2010). A number of these methods are indicative of the cognitive and emotional rebuilding that takes place after our 'assumptive world' (Parkes 1971) has been breached through trauma; a process referred to as 'rumination' (Tedeschi et al. 2015).

Tedeschi and colleagues purport that in the aftermath of the event rumination often occurs on an intrusive basis as negative thoughts, memories and imagery spontaneously present in our conscious awareness. Overtime, rumination can occur on a more deliberate basis, where the processing of memories is intentionally undertaken in order to make sense and find meaning (Tedeschi et al. 2015). In the women's narratives, these conscious contemplations (such as through birth discussions with maternity professionals) were often 'upsetting' and 'deeply distressing' but also, as reflected by Janet, operated as the basis through which new beliefs, assumptions and growth could be attained:

[I]t turned my feelings of failure into anger. It enabled me to deal with it and move on.

(Thomson 2007, 255)

These strategies, as indicated by Janet, appeared to enable women to emotionally and cognitively reframe their traumatic birth and empowered them to feel in control over what was to come. Diane described how she 'wouldn't let it happen the second time round, I was not prepared to let it' (Thomson 2007, 261). The women's determination to succeed represents the positive force of growth; as indicated in the following quote by Ruth, it reflected a force which required them to accept their former trials and to have the courage to face a future ordeal:

I think with X [second birth], I felt that I'd done everything I possibly could to prepare for it. I accepted that it was unknown what was going to happen and everything, but I'd done everything that I could to make it the best experience I could.

(Thomson 2007, 260)

A further key area of growth in the women's accounts is how they developed 'trust' in their bodies and capabilities. For some, as described by a mother in Beck and Watson's (2010) study, this new knowledge was an empowering, life-affirming experience:

Toward the end of pregnancy, I did the birth art exercises out of the book *Birthing from Within* … I began to trust myself. That will stay with me forever. This is more than just what I needed to birth the way I wanted to. That is what I needed to become a real woman.

(Beck and Watson 2010, 246)

Relating to others

As other chapters in this book have highlighted repeatedly, relationality and connectedness are central to interpretations of spiritual wellbeing. This is no less true than in PTG as concerns related to positive changes in interpersonal relationships, both within and outside of personal networks, are significant.

Following a traumatic birth some women described a heightened level of vigilance and protectiveness over their infants. For example, they referred to using constant surveillance, extended breastfeeding and bed-sharing as a means to 'protect' their infants from further harm (Thomson 2007). These maternal behaviours were often initiated to compensate for the guilt and self-blame associated with the birth, and their emotional unavailability in the early post-natal period (Thomson 2007, Beck and Watson 2010). However, they also held growth potential through forming positive attachment relationships and becoming what they considered to be a good mother by 'doing the right thing' (Thomson 2007, 243). For others, the shared nature of trauma between them and their babies served to magnify their attachment relationship. Diane claimed to love her baby 'even more' due to their mutual harrowing experience:

> I think maybe in some way it kind of made me love her more because to me she'd been through a lot of trauma as well, the first thing she experiences of life is something grabbing hold of her head and yanking her out.
>
> *(Thomson 2007, 226)*

Women in Beck and Watson's study (2016) referred to how a traumatic birth had strengthened their relationships with the infant born through trauma as well as their older children. One reported how it had become crucial for her children to 'know love, to know they are delighted in, to feel safe, to feel empowered and supported, and to feel nurtured' (Beck and Watson 2016, 268). Women emphasised a need to be a positive role model for their children, especially their daughters (Beck and Watson 2016).

A traumatic birth is often an alienating experience where women feel unable or unwilling to disclose their negative emotions (Fenech and Thomson 2014). However, in the study by Beck and Watson (2016) some referred to how the birth had led them to have stronger relationships with their partners. One woman described how the opportunity to discuss the harrowing and 'gruesome' details of the birth had provided a new 'relationship nakedness' – where she felt secure enough to openly disclose her innermost thoughts and feelings, which in turn enabled them to have a deeper level of connection (Beck and Watson 2016, 268).

A further area of growth was evident through women being able to hold intimate discussions with friends and others about the birth (such as via birth trauma websites/social networks) (Thomson 2007, Beck and Watson 2016). As reflected in Clare's story, these opportunities were important to validate and normalise their experiences as well as enabling them to develop new and more meaningful relationships:

> There's similar themes and words that … you can relate to and that in itself has been really really helpful beyond anything, talking to other mums that really understand because they've been through it, they know exactly what you mean when you say things even though everybody's story's really different.
>
> *(Thomson 2007, 304)*

The women in Beck and Watson's (2016) study who worked within healthcare described more positive relationships with their patients. Other mothers also referred to how their own adversity had provided them with a deepened sense of empathy for others who may face a similar situation (Thomson 2007, Beck and Watson 2016). Jackie, for example, demonstrates how she was now able to appreciate the negative implications of receiving midwifery care aligned with interventions, rather than normality:

> I've a few friends who are pregnant now for the first time and … I'd hate for them to go through a similar experience [to] what I went through so you really want to reinforce don't listen to midwives, each intervention leads to something else, try and keep active, positions and things like that, really shouldn't be down to someone like me to do it but you'd just hate for them to go to hospital and lie in a bed and [the] same things to happen unnecessarily.
>
> *(Thomson 2007, 357)*

Although Jackie's perspective on midwives appears damning it needs to be understood in the context of her experience of childbirth and need not infer universal experience of midwifery care.

New possibilities

The final domain concerns new interests or opportunities that are available or desirable following a traumatic life event. This gestures the openness to possibilities previously unknown and appreciated indicating perhaps women's emergent spiritual wellbeing and growth.

In the women's narratives these new possibilities often signified altruistic behaviours and new life trajectories. Some women joined a birth theatre group, which involved acting out their traumatic birth experiences at academic and professional events (i.e. workshops, training events, conferences) (Thomson 2007). Others referred to how they wanted to, or were, providing support via online forums to empower women (Thomson 2007, Beck and Watson 2016). Holly decides to engage in these activities based on a desire to protect others from having the same experience, as well as to offer support to those who suffered a similar fate:

> When X [consultant midwife] offered us these things to do [i.e. join a birth theatre group, to meet other women], to help other women, [it] made me more strong to do something, to help other people not to have to go through that and to understand that things can be different.
>
> *(Thomson 2007, 366)*

Examples of reaching out to others reveals a need to give back and support others in different ways. One woman in the Beck and Watson (2016) study had established and volunteered at a local International Caesarean Awareness Network, and another (who had a midwifery background) provided voluntary support at a crisis pregnancy centre. Others embarked on new careers through study in nursing, midwifery and child and family health areas (Beck and Watson 2016). One described how her subsequent nursing degree had enabled her to address her former adversity and to develop inner strength:

> I then went to the university to complete a nursing degree. I faced a number of fears in my nursing placements. As I did this I became stronger and stronger and after a lot of hard work I achieved my Bachelor of Health Science in Nursing.
>
> *(Beck and Watson 2016, 269)*

Extending one's reach of influence to others beyond one's own personal life speaks of connectedness to community and an altruistic tendency born of experiences. This quality of compassion towards others is another example of spirituality manifesting among the women in these studies.

Spirituality and PTG

Spirituality as religion, as well as how spirituality concerns the meaning and purpose of life events, connectedness to others and self-transcendence are all reported in the nursing and health literature (Callister and Khalaf 2010). This chapter has revealed how spirituality is strongly associated with PTG due to how times of crisis create an impetus for deep spiritual beliefs and renewed life meanings (Murray and Zentner 1989).

Some women referred to how their experience of trauma had created 'transpersonal connectedness' with a higher being/God (Greenstreet 2006, 11) – an event that led to self-transcendence through renewed and deeper religious beliefs. The 'interconnectedness' and capacity for meaningful relationships associated with spirituality (Lyall 2000) was also reflected through women forming more positive relationships with their children and partners, and the valued connections formed with others who had suffered a similar experience. Women also developed higher order spiritual meanings through new purpose and significance in their life-worlds (Greenstreet 2006). They reported feeling blessed for having a healthy infant, more appreciative of the pleasure and love they received from their family members, and how the experience of trauma had created an impetus to adopt positive maternal behaviours.

Spirituality concerns structures of significance that give meaning and directions to our lives (Lyall 2000). In the women's accounts, they referred to how they now held new life-meanings through the use of altruistic and benevolent behaviours in their daily interactions as well as via new volunteer and career opportunities. Their new knowledge represented 'a life wisdom' (Linley 2003) – a deeper level of understanding and meaning of the significance of birth, and how women wanted to use this knowledge to empower others. Finally, the spiritual components of renewed belief and faith in self (Greenstreet 2006, Lyall 2000) are revealed in the women's inner strength, conviction and 'trust' in their capabilities to face further adversities (i.e. childbirth) following an experience of trauma.

Implications for practice and research

Tedeschi and colleagues posit that it is primarily through deliberate ruminations that PTG is possible. Suggestions to facilitate deep reflection and to elicit areas of growth are offered, as follows:

- Currently routine debriefing is not recommended within current UK guidance (National Institute of Health and Clinical Excellence 2006). However, the possibility for women to be offered a 'birth reflection' meeting that includes the processing of cognitive, emotional and spiritual elements related to their childbirth experience should be considered.
- Maternity healthcare professionals are considered to be in a prime position to promote PTG following childbirth. Tedeschi et al. (2015) recommend that when working with those who have experienced a traumatic event, professionals should adopt the role of an 'expert companion'. This approach involves active and effective listening, respecting and validating the individual's subjective experience of the event, and assisting the individual to identify salient areas of growth.
- Opportunities for women to discuss their experiences within a mutually supportive network of women, such as through postnatal support groups, or available services/organisation, e.g. Birth Trauma Association. Women could also be encouraged to write journals or engage in expressive writing (Ullrich and Lutgendorf 2002).
- A further strategy could be to share stories of growth with other women, to provide optimism that renewal is possible.

While PTG has been studied following a variety of challenging life situations, it is under-researched in relation to a traumatic birth. Further qualitative and/ or mixed method studies to focus on how growth is experienced should be undertaken. As childbirth is a significant life event, with elements of PTG identified irrespective of how women internalise the event (e.g. Sawyer and Ayers 2009, Sawyer et al. 2012), studies could compare the level and degrees of growth among women with different birth appraisals (i.e. positive or traumatic). PTSD onset among those in attendance (i.e. partners, health professionals) at a traumatic/difficult/complex birth are areas of increasing interest (e.g. Sheen, Spiby and Slade 2015). Research to explore the positive outcomes of these experiences, and the potential for practice development could prove illuminating. Finally, interventions designed to encourage rumination and to assess the impact of such on PTG, emotional adversity and spiritual distress should be considered.

Conclusion

A traumatic birth is a deeply distressing event, with negative implications for women, infants and family members. However, through drawing on the PTG and spirituality literature I have highlighted how a traumatic birth – normal or medicalised – can lead to growth and renewal. These insights 'de-massify' the current dichotomies of what constitutes a 'good' birth and emphasise the importance of subjective interpretations. They also offer a more salutogenic perspective to identify the positive implications of a traumatic birth for women and others. While the obvious ideal is to prevent trauma from occurring in the first place, the findings in the studies mentioned here highlight how women were able to form deeper spiritual understandings, feel more connected and enjoy improved meaningful relationships, personal strength, direction towards new life meanings and purpose. While the co-existence of negative emotions associated with a traumatic birth is inevitable, the traditional approach to such morbidities (such as PTSD) is problem-orientated, with interventions designed to maintain baseline wellbeing. Opportunities for rumination, to enable women to re-assimilate their memories and to identify areas of growth thereby offer new and healing potential.

References

American Psychiatric Association (APA). 2013. *Diagnostic and Statistical Manual of Mental Disorders: Fifth Edition*. Arlington, VA: APA.

Antonovsky, A. 1979. *Health, stress and coping*. San Francisco, CA: Jossey-Bass.

Ayers, S., Bond, R., Bertullies, S. and Wijma, K. 2016. "The aetiology of post-traumatic stress following childbirth: a meta-analysis and theoretical framework." *Psychological Medicine* 46 (6): 1121–1134.

Beck, C.T. and Watson, S. 2010. "Subsequent childbirth after a previous traumatic birth." *Nursing Research* 59: 241–49.

Beck, C.T. and Watson, S. 2016. "Posttraumatic growth following birth trauma: 'I was broken. Now I am Unbreakable.'" *MCN: American Journal of Maternal Child Nursing* 1 (5): 264–271.

Black, B.P. and Sandelowski, M. 2010. "Personal growth after severe fetal diagnosis." *Western Journal of Nursing Research* 32 (8): 1011–1030.

Black, B.P. and Wright, P. 2012. "Posttraumatic growth and transformation as outcomes of perinatal loss." *Illness, Crisis & Loss* 20 (3): 225–237.

Calhoun, L.G. and Tedeschi, R.G. 1998. "Posttraumatic growth: Future directions." In *Posttraumatic growth: Positive change in the aftermath of crisis*, edited by Richard G. Tedeschi, Crystal L. Park and Lawrence G. Calhoun, 215–238. Mahwah, NJ: Lawrence Erlbaum Associates.

Callister, L.C. and Khalaf, I. 2010. "Spirituality in childbearing women." *Journal of Perinatal Education* 19 (2): 16–24.

Crowther, S., Smythe, L. and Spence, D. 2014. "Mood and birth experience." *Women and Birth* 27: 21–25.

Davis-Floyd, R. 1992. *Birth as an American rite of passage*. Berkeley and Los Angeles, CA: University of California Press.

Downe, S. and McCourt, C. 2004. "From being to becoming: Reconstructing childbirth knowledge." In *Normal Childbirth Evidence and Debate,* edited by Soo Downe, 3–24. China: Churchill Livingstone.

Elmir, R., Schmied, V., Wilkes, L. and Jackson, D. 2010. "Women's perceptions and experiences of a traumatic birth: A meta-ethnography." *Journal of Advanced Nursing* 66: 2142–2153. DOI: 10.1111/j.1365-2648.2010.05391.x.

Fenech, G. and Thomson, G. 2014. "'Tormented by ghosts of their past': A meta-synthesis to explore the psychosocial implications of a traumatic birth on maternal wellbeing." *Midwifery* 30: 185–93.

Frost, J., Pope, C., Liebling, R. and Murphy, D. 2006. "Utopian birth and the discourse of natural birth." *Social Theory & Health* 4: 299–318.

Gaskin, I.M. 1990. *Spiritual midwifery: Third Edition.* Summertown, TN: The Book Publishing Company.

Greenstreet, W. 2006. *Integrating spirituality in health and social care: Perspectives and practical approaches.* Oxford: Radcliffe Publishing.

Hunter, B. and Warren, L. 2014. "Midwives' experiences of workplace resilience." *Midwifery* 30 (8): 926–34.

Janoff-Bulman, R. 1992. *Shattered assumptions. Towards a new psychology of trauma.* New York: The Free Press.

Linley, P.A. 2003. "Positive adaptation to trauma: Wisdom as both process and outcome." *Journal of Traumatic Stress* 16 (6): 601–10.

Lyall, D. 2000. "Spiritual institutions." In *Spirituality in Health Care Contexts,* edited by Helen Orchard, 47–56. London: Jessica Kingsley Publishers.

Mauger, B. 2000. *Reclaiming the spirituality of birth.* Ireland: Collins Press.

Mautner, E., Stern, C., Deutsch, M., Nagele, E., Greimel, E., Lang, U. and Cervar-Zivkovic, M. 2013. "The impact of resilience on psychological outcomes in women after preeclampsia: an observational cohort study." *Health and Quality of Life Outcomes* 14 (11): 194. doi: 10.1186/1477-7525-11-194.

Murray, R. and Zentner, J. 1989. *Nursing concepts for health promotion.* London: Prentice Hall.

National Institute of Clinical Excellence. 2006. *Postnatal care up to 8 weeks after birth.* London: NICE.

Parkes, C.M. 1971. "Psycho-social transitions: A field for study." *Social Science & Medicine* 5: 101–115.

Peterson, G. 1996. "Childbirth: The ordinary miracle: Effects of devaluation of childbirth on women's self-esteem and family relationships." *Journal of Prenatal and Perinatal Psychology and Health* 11 (2): 101–109.

Ryding, E.L., Lukasse, M., Parys, A.S.V., Wangel, A.M., Karro, H., Kristjansdottir, H., Schroll, A.M. and Schei, B. 2015. "Fear of childbirth and risk of cesarean delivery: A cohort study in six European countries." *Birth* 42 (1): 48–55.

Sawyer, A. and Ayers, S. 2009. "Post-traumatic growth in women after childbirth." *Psychology and Health* 24 (4): 457–471.

Sawyer, A., Ayers, S., Young, D., Bradley, R. and Smith, H., 2012. "Posttraumatic growth after childbirth: A prospective study." *Psychology & health* 27 (3): 362–377.

Sawyer, A., Nakić Radoš, S., Ayers, S. and Burn, E., 2015. "Personal growth in UK and Croatian women following childbirth: A preliminary study." *Journal of Reproductive and Infant Psychology* 33 (3): 294–307.

Shakespeare-Finch, J. and Lurie-Beck, J. 2014. "A meta-analytic clarification of the relationship between posttraumatic growth and symptoms of posttraumatic distress disorder." *Journal of Anxiety Disorders* 28 (2): 223–229.

Sheen, K., Spiby, H. and Slade, P. 2015. "Exposure to traumatic perinatal experiences and posttraumatic stress symptoms in midwives: Prevalence and association with burnout." *International Journal of Nursing Studies* 52 (2): 578–587.

Stoll, K., Hall, W., Janssen, P. and Carty, E. 2014. "Why are young Canadians afraid of birth? A survey study of childbirth fear and birth preferences among Canadian University students." *Midwifery* 30 (2): 220–226.

Tanyi, R.A. 2002. "Towards clarification of the meaning of spirituality." *Journal of Advanced Nursing* 39 (5): 500–509.

Tedeschi, R.G. and Calhoun, L.G. 1995. *Trauma and transformation: Growing in the aftermath of suffering.* Thousand Oaks, CA: Sage.

Tedeschi, R.G. and Calhoun, L.G. 1996. "The Posttraumatic Growth Inventory: Measuring the positive legacy of trauma." *Journal of Traumatic Stress* 9: 455–472.

Tedeschi, R.G. and Calhoun, L.G. 2004. *Posttraumatic growth: Conceptual foundation and empirical evidence.* Philadelphia, PA: Lawrence Erlbaum Associates.

Tedeschi, R.G., Calhoun, L.G. and Groleau, J.M. 2015. "Clinical applications of posttraumatic growth." In *Positive psychology in practice: Promoting human flourishing in work, health, education, and everyday life, 2nd edition,* edited by Stephen Joseph, 503–518. New Jersey: John Wiley & Sons.

Tedeschi, R.G., Park, C.L. and Calhoun, L.G. 1998. *Posttraumatic growth: Positive changes in the aftermath of crisis.* Mahwah, NJ: Erlbaum.

Thomson, G. 2007. "*A hero's tale of childbirth: An interpretive phenomenological study of traumatic and positive childbirth.*" Unpublished doctoral dissertation. UK: University of Central Lancashire.

Thomson, G. and Downe, S. 2008. "Widening the trauma discourse: the link between childbirth and experiences of abuse." *Journal of Psychosomatic Obstetrics & Gynaecology* 29 (4): 268–273.

Thomson, G. and Downe, S. 2010. "Changing the future to change the past: Women's experiences of a positive birth following a traumatic birth experience." *Journal of Reproductive and Infant Psychology* 28 (1): 102–112.

Thomson, G. and Downe, S. 2013. "A hero's tale of childbirth." *Midwifery* 29 (7): 765–771.

Turkstra, E., Gamble, J., Creedy, D.K., Fenwick, J., Barclay, L., Buist, A., Ryding, E.L. and Scuffham, P.A. 2013. "PRIME; impact of previous mental health problems on health related quality of life in women with childbirth trauma." *Archives of Women's Mental Health* 16: 561–564.

Ullrich, P.M. and Lutgendorf, S.K. 2002. "Journaling about stressful events: effects of cognitive processing and emotional expression." *Annals of Behaviour Medicine* 24 (3): 244–250.

Zadoroznyj, M. 1999. "Social class, social selves and social control in childbirth." *Sociology of Health and Illness* 21 (3): 267–289.

11

SPIRITUALITY WHEN A NEWBORN IS UNWELL

Sílvia Caldeira

Introduction

Parents usually place high expectations on their pregnancy journey and having a successful birth. From the beginning of the desire to be parents, the idea of a 'normal' and 'healthy' pregnancy starts arising in the thoughts, in the heart and in the soul of the parents. Sometimes this is not possible and the pregnancy comes to an end with an early delivery and the birth of an unwell baby who is different from the expected baby and is living with different conditions. In these situations parents may start a grieving journey involving deep and intimate feelings, based on denial or anger. Healthcare professionals are in a privileged position of proximity alongside parents coping with these circumstances and can help guarantee both human support and to promote resilience. In these suffering moments parents often turn to their belief systems seeking strength, conversely some religious (or otherwise) believers start questioning their faith. A child is often a significant part of the couple's meaning and also part of the individual meaning in life. The whole process of having an unwell child can be a time of suffering and be lived as a profound spiritual experience which is frequently transformative in many aspects.

This chapter will discuss opportunities for a spiritual approach that should be taken by the healthcare team, because these situations are mostly spiritual in nature – that is, these situations often involve questioning the meaning in life while turning into a reflexive journey about self-identity and life expectations. The spiritual needs of parents and the baby when the baby is unwell following birth in a neonatal unit and issues around the baby will be discussed. In addition, the role of the multidisciplinary healthcare team concerning the issues around the grieving journey and the recognition of spiritual distress are considered as a state of suffering related to the impaired ability to experience meaning in life through connectedness with self, others, world, or a Superior Being (Caldeira, Carvalho and Vieira 2013).

A FICTIONAL CASE STUDY

Sarah and Paul have been married for seven years. Both were born in the 1970s and are Catholic. Since the day they got married they dreamed about having three children. After two years of marriage they realised that Sarah was not able to get pregnant. They submitted themselves to several fertility treatments and had a baby after a five-year journey. In the 32nd week of pregnancy baby Mary was unexpectedly born, and Sarah and Paul were, suddenly, premature parents. The day after the birth, they were informed about how critical their baby's health was. Nurse Angelica stood near the incubator with Sarah and Paul and observed that Paul was crying while asking: 'Oh God, why is this happening to us after so long, after such a suffering journey?' His wife, Sarah, was hugging him and praying. In this moment nurse Angelica kept her presence in silence.

Learning from Mary, Sarah, Paul and Angelica

Mary: spiritual reflections from an unwell baby

In the fictional case study above, Mary represents all unwell premature babies. These babies are those who are born before 28 weeks of gestational age (extremely preterm), between 28 and 32 weeks (very preterm), or between 32 and 37 weeks (moderate to late preterm) (World Health Organization 2012, Blencowe et al. 2013). So, an infant is considered to be premature when born less than 37 weeks, while an infant born between 37 and 42 weeks is considered full term. More than one in 10 babies are born preterm, affecting many families all around the world, and these rates are rising (World Health Organization 2012, Blencowe et al. 2013). As a result of this trend an international agenda focused on research and health policies is emerging. The presence of these babies is challenging science and technology, but also leading to ethical discussions concerning viability and clinical decision-making, for both professionals and parents (Schroeder 2008). It is vital to keep in mind that healthcare providers are not absent from moral distress and are committed and affected in such decisions (Cavaliere et al. 2010).

Premature babies are physically different from term babies and may easily represent vulnerability. The size, the skin, the body proportions are different, and looking at a premature baby for the first time could promote emotion due to their fragile condition (Hwang et al. 2013, Ribeiro et al. 2015, Bélanger-Lévesque et al. 2016). Premature babies thus provide an opportunity to look at being human through the lenses of dignity and respect for such vulnerability and human nature. Dignity of vulnerable babies should be taken into account as it is in other contexts of care, such as in elderly care (Reed et al. 2003). This is an interesting lesson to take from these babies, particularly to healthcare providers who are expected to guarantee that their clinical practice is grounded in values and ethical principles based on respect for human life (International Council of Nurses 2012). An unwell newborn needs complete care; they are totally dependent on another human to keep living. The vulnerability of an unwell newborn represents an opportunity for compassionate care that preserves the dignity of the newborn. Additionally, we are charged with 'being in the moment' and 'emotional connection', both of which have been found to be aspects of compassionate care (Christiansen et al. 2015), relevant in these situations of profound vulnerability.

For parents, these babies are bringing a unique opportunity for love and the need for love is one of the core spiritual needs (McSherry and Smith 2012). Spirituality has been considered a dimension of the human being, and spiritual needs are particularly relevant in times of crisis and illness (Baldacchino and Draper 2001, McSherry 2006, Weathers, McCarthy and Coffey 2016). This dimension is particularly important in health and is often defined as the search for meaning in life, transcendence and connectedness (Weathers, McCarthy and Coffey 2016). Thus, spirituality could be understood as an exclusive dimension of the adult, as it seems to be based on the ability of being aware of self and living circumstances. But the newborn should also be considered a human being, having a spiritual nature and spiritual needs (Caldeira and Hall 2012).

The age and the developmental stage of a person seem to be critical in relation to their understanding or expression of religiosity and spirituality, particularly in children and adolescents (Smith and McSherry 2004). Regardless of the absence of awareness and transcendence, baby Mary, who is metaphorically representing all unwell newborns, has the unfailing power of connection with those who love her and those who provide care for her. Mary seems to personify an unequal transforming capacity in the lives of those around her. There is a 'before' Mary and an 'after' Mary, no matter the health condition, for it is mainly her presence and life. This is the most transformative and spiritual aspect that babies are bringing, first, to their parents and, also and consequently, to healthcare providers. The baby is promoting a spiritually awakened opportunity and this has been considered an important experience regardless the age of the child (Fosareli 2012).

These experiences are hard to describe in words and are usually expressed in the sense of feelings, which are more intuitive than cognitive (Fosareli 2012). Babies reflect the sacredness of life and evoke respect, love and compassion, which are the pillars of spirituality in this context (Figure 11.1).

Sarah and Paul: spiritual reflections from the parents' experience

In the case study at the start of this chapter, Sarah and Paul represent all parents, regardless the gender. Parenthood has been considered an important transition in making existential meaning (Prinds et al. 2013). The birth of a premature or

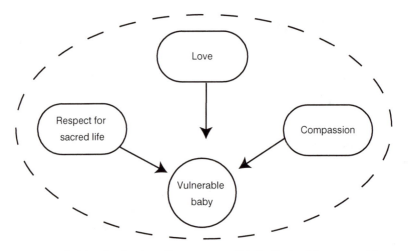

FIGURE 11.1 Spiritual reflections from an unwell baby for healthcare providers and family

unwell baby in a critical condition often places parents in stressful situations due to physiological conditions and psychological problems inherent to this situational transition. Emotional distress, depression, anxiety, guilt and grief have been identified as some experiences and feelings of mothers while living this transition. Spirituality has been widely described as a significant dimension during life transitions and illness and defined as:

> a way of being in the world in which a person feels a sense of connectedness to self, others, and/or a higher power or nature; a sense of meaning in life; and transcendence beyond self, everyday living, and suffering.
>
> *(Weathers, McCarthy and Coffey 2016, 93)*

When facing their baby in such a critical health condition, parents are living a loss of the baby they were waiting for. The baby's physical poor condition, the technological environment and the nurses taking such an important role in providing care may promote a sense of distress and suffering. Spirituality was shown to act as a coping resource, particularly useful in difficult situations (Callister and Khalaf 2010). But spirituality is also important in daily life and only emerges in un-ordinary and challenging situations. Such experiences provide a deep dimension that connects us to an 'intensification of the human' experience and can disclose a positive dimension to life (Bélanger-Lévesque et al. 2016). This is a critical idea when discussing spirituality in children or in childbirth. Considering that health is no longer the absence of illness but a whole sense of wellbeing, in all human dimensions, including spiritualty then, the spiritual dimension of childbirth could be also turned into a health promotion opportunity for the healthcare teams and midwives in particular.

Research about the spiritual dimension in childbirth is quite poor when compared to end-of-life care in older people or in the context of palliative care. But some studies and discussions have been published exploring pediatrics, neonatology (Caldeira and Hall 2012), childbirth (Crowther and Hall 2015), pediatric intensive care units (Nascimento et al. 2016), or adolescents (Büssing et al. 2010, Taylor et al. 2015). The need for an evidence based practice in health and also for translational research in healthcare contexts should drive the enthusiasm and motivation to improve research into spirituality concerning issues in and around childbirth (Crowther and Hall 2015).

Evidence from a mixed methods comparative study exploring a neonatal intensive care unit revealed how the experience of mothers and fathers is intense (Bélanger-Lévesque et al. 2016). The study found similar themes from both mothers and fathers such as respect, moral responsibility, beauty of life, gratitude, greater than self and prayer. But when comparing the scoring of themes between mothers and fathers differences were found between fragility of life, self-accomplishment, meaningfulness and letting go (Bélanger-Lévesque et al. 2016). This reflects other earlier studies. Mothers often describe feelings of fear, guilt, anxiety, suffering, searching for meaning, hope and being concerned about the suffering or pain of the newborn (Gale et al. 2004, Ribeiro et al. 2015).

These emotional aspects are similar to spiritual needs listed in the literature; meaning and purpose, need for love and harmonious relationships, need for forgiveness, need for a source of hope and strength, need for trust, need for expression of personal beliefs and values and need for spiritual practices (which may include religiosity) (McSherry and Smith 2012). Parents' experiences demonstrate aspects of the spiritual dimension within the Neonatal Intensive Care Unit (NICU), which is mostly explored in its physical, technological and psychosocial aspects. This is a challenge for healthcare professionals, particularly nurses and/or midwives who are providing care to parents and babies.

A study about the experience of fathers in the NICU found two main themes: the father-baby approach and remaining in the NICU (overcoming obstacles and revealing motivations), and the father being included in the care of the preterm child (limits and possibilities) (Soares et al. 2016). When looking at these themes it is possible to find small but valuable insights about how we can provide holistic, human and spiritual care, which promotes meaning making in this situation and sense of fulfilment. Fathers often keep working if there are no other children. Often fathers take an important role in keeping the routines as normal as possible for siblings who are also in a dynamic and transitional process. Holism is a crucial concept not only in healthcare care delivery but also in the approach to the family as a unit that works together because a family is dynamic and as a whole is different from the sum of the parts. Parents, for example, felt constraints imposed by the routine of the institution, the obligations and need to keep working and missing paternity leave (Soares et al. 2016).

Sarah and Paul are representing all couples, regardless the gender, that are living this stressful situation. They are enclosed in a grieving journey, which often starts with the sense of losing the expected baby and all those parenthood experiences they have been imagined to come through. Grieving is an individual response to loss and is influenced by many factors: physical, emotional, occupational, social, intellectual and spiritual (Dyer 2005). The spiritual aspects of grieving often comprise doubting their belief system; questioning spiritual values; experiencing spiritual injury; loss of faith; disappointment in religion, clergy and church members; feeling betrayed by God or spiritual force, angry with God or deity; and being concerned with their own death (Dyer 2005) (see Figure 11.2). While experiencing grief parents are looking for answers, explanations and understanding. Sometimes they blame others, God or themselves for what is happening, as they need time to understand and accept the situation. The NICU represents, in many cases, a spiritual environment (Caldeira and Hall 2012). When expressing suffering, distress, anger towards God or beliefs, parents are appealing for support in this journey. Healthcare providers should be aware of and attend to these needs aiming to promote resilience, wellbeing and supporting in a meaning-making process. These are the pillars of spiritual care, which are explored in the next section.

Nurse Angelica: understanding and implementing spiritual care

Nurse Angelica was present and therefore shared the deep, intimate and suffering episode when Sarah and Paul were looking at baby Mary, just after being informed about her critical health status. In the fictional case study at the start of this chapter, Angelica represents nurses and/or midwives who often

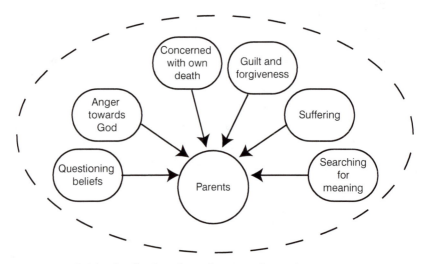

FIGURE 11.2 Spiritual reflections from the parents' experience

deal with these painful situations in their clinical practice. But also, the other healthcare members within the multidisciplinary team, who are daily attending people in suffering in NICU, where the family (parents and baby) should take the core position within the caring process.

Nurses in NICU may experience difficult situations and moral distress related to the ethically challenging care they provide (Cavaliere et al. 2010, Kain 2007, Almeida, Moraes and Cunha 2016). The caring experiences around loss and birth affect healthcare providers, whether a premature delivery, unwell newborn or stillbirth. For example, consultants describe stillbirth as a very difficult experience characterised by carrying a burden (Nuzum, Meaney and O'Donoghue 2014, 2016). Nurses' emotional overload has been also identified in an integrative literature review about the perceptions of nursing care in neonatology (Ribeiro et al. 2015). Interestingly, a recent study with neonatal nurses in Australia about a hypothetical premature birth situation concluded that nurses, if in a similar condition, would not choose to resuscitate and provide care to their own babies as they do to the other babies they are caring for of 24 or less weeks of age, taking into account their own caring experiences (Green et al. 2016). On many occasions these babies are in palliative care conditions, but few guidelines have been defined to integrate palliative care in NICU (Mancini et al. 2014), and little is known about effective implementation. Race, poverty and difficulties in healthcare provision seems to be risk factors for pregnancy complications, and this is an example of the need for effective palliative care services, which would be appropriate to patients particular needs (Boss and Clarke-Pounder 2012). Recently, the American Academy of Pediatrics defined pediatric palliative care goals, which included the improvement of children's quality and enjoyment of life while helping families to adapt and function during the illness and through bereavement; facilitating informed decision making by patients, families and healthcare professionals; and assisting with ongoing coordination of care among clinicians and across various sites of care (Section on Hospice and Palliative Medicine and Committee on Hospital Care 2013). Palliative care is dignity-preserving care, while promoting, supporting and searching for meaning in illness situations is often deeply spiritual. Spirituality is a critical dimension of palliative care, and this is particularly important in NICU or in caring for an unwell newborn, as the grieving process should be supported from the beginning to beyond and after death.

Spirituality, as a coping mechanism, promotes a sense of serenity and peace not only for parents but also for nurses, as those who were not spiritual scored higher levels of spiritual distress than those who described themselves as very or somewhat spiritual (Cavaliere et al. 2010). Nurses often recognise their role in providing spiritual care, as this is included in a holistic paradigm of care. But nurses and midwives often recognise feeling underprepared and feel that they lack the competencies or guidelines in providing spiritual care (Van Leeuwen and Cusveller 2004, Baldacchinho 2006, Attard, Baldacchino and Camilleri 2014). In fact, no unique set of competencies and guidelines has been agreed to inform spiritual care. Spiritual care is a concept and a complex intervention that merges health knowledge and other disciplines providing the foundations for understanding the human spirit and condition and needs to occur as a multidisciplinary approach. Spiritual care cannot be confined to purely a professional defined service as it arises within human encounters requiring both skill and humility of its practitioners (Rumbold 2012).

The understanding of spiritual care and the limits for nursing and midwifery intervention within the multidisciplinary healthcare team are not always as clear as expected, and so nurses may consider chaplains to be the main responsible professional for providing spiritual care, especially if spirituality is confined exclusively to religiosity. This could be reductionist, and those parents who are not believers of a recognised faith may have spiritual needs that need to be addressed by others, not only by clergy or chaplains.

A recent concept analysis of spiritual care identified seven attributes: healing presence, therapeutic use of self, intuitive sense, exploration of the spiritual perspective, patient-centeredness, meaning-centred therapeutic intervention and creation of a spiritually nurturing environment (Ramezani et al. 2014). These attributes highlight the 'doing' dimension of spiritual care that is often considered a way of 'being' – thus, difficult to perform and time consuming. Time has been considered a barrier in providing spiritual care, but when we embrace the meaningfulness of each moment of care it becomes evident that time need not be considered a barrier. There are many significant opportunities in supporting spiritual wellbeing and meaning making whilst providing care (Caldeira and Timmins 2015). The attributes of spiritual care are related to communication and healthcare professional and patient relationship. In the context of NICU the healthcare team has the opportunity and privilege of being in close proximity with parents and this requires therapeutic or effective relationships based on communication skills. Healthcare teams should therefore keep a patient-centred approach, and each professional (medical, nursing and midwifery) should be aware of their important individual role in making all care effective and meaningful. In particular, nurses and midwives should be aware and develop the competencies for spiritual care (Van Leeuwen and Cusveller 2004, Baldacchinho 2006, Attard, Baldacchino and Camilleri 2014).

Despite there being no agreed competency checklist for spiritual care there are recognised broad components comprising: the awareness and use of self; the spiritual dimension of the nursing process; and assurance and quality of expertise and ethical aspects of care (Van Leeuwen and Cusveller 2004, Baldacchinho 2006, Attard, Baldacchino and Camilleri 2014). Again, the first component relates to the use of a nurse's personal skills and experience. Nurses' experiences and expertise or professional maturity seems to influence the provision of spiritual care and to the relationship with patients (Giske and Cone 2015). The second component relates to the nursing process, driven from the assessment, the diagnosis, the planning of the interventions and the evaluation of the outcomes. This is a clinical reasoning process, also used by nurses who deal with spirituality in clinical practice (Caldeira et al. 2016, 2017) (see Figure 11.3). The third

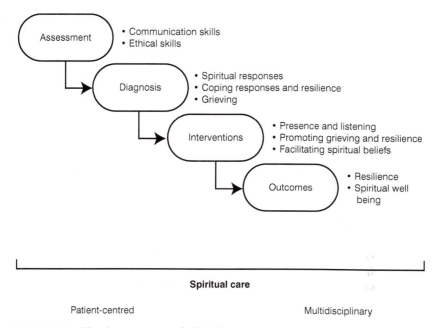

FIGURE 11.3   Nursing process and clinical reasoning

component underlines the ethical aspects of spiritual care. Additionally, in the NICU context, these should be taken into account, namely, the awareness of competencies to provide spiritual care and the referral to the best healthcare professional to address parents' needs. Within the healthcare team, nurses are more often near the baby and parents in the NICU. The closeness of the relationship with the nurse is a core element in delivering spiritual care.

As explained previously, spirituality is broader than religiosity, and nurses should be aware of this when assessing parents' spirituality and when providing spiritual care. Being religious or not, nurses can transform their presence into a healing presence, and this means that parents may feel the nurses' empathy, compassion and commitment in transforming suffering in meaningful moments in their lives. Spiritual assessment should be grounded in trust and in a well-established relationship. Nurses should use their senses to assess all that they can observe, feel and listen. Sometimes being present is all that parents need in these times of crisis. To assess spirituality nurses should observe mothers, rituals, objects or requests.

On many occasions parents ask for permission to keep a religious object near the baby. This may constitute the first connection with nurses to explore spirituality, beliefs and coping. Using these strategies, nurses are creating a spiritually nurturing environment, exploring spiritual perspective and, at the same time, providing a healing presence. During these moments nurses assess spiritual wellbeing, sources of hope, strength and meaning, and coping resources. Having this information, nurses may then use professional classifications to support their diagnosis and the planning of interventions. For example, NANDA International (NANDA-I) is an international classification of nursing diagnoses and integrates diagnoses related to spirituality, spiritual wellbeing and spiritual distress (Herdman and Kamitsuru 2014). This classification is dynamic and nursing research is helpful in testing the accuracy of the diagnoses that are listed. Spiritual distress is a diagnosis that has been included in NANDA-I classification since 1978, and is defined as

> a state of suffering related to the impaired ability to experience the meaning of life by connecting with self, others, or a Higher Being.
>
> *(Herdman and Kamitsuru 2014, 372)*

Other nursing diagnoses related to spirituality include 'risk for spiritual distress', 'readiness for enhanced spiritual wellbeing', 'impaired religiosity', readiness for enhanced religiosity', and 'risk for impaired religiosity'. Other diagnoses could also be taken into account when assessing spirituality, such as 'death anxiety', 'grieving', 'impaired resilience' or 'disabled family coping'. The classifications include the risk factors, related factors and defining characteristics according to the diagnosis, and these are invaluable in reaching the most accurate diagnosis. Classifications are not prescriptive and not exclusive for clinical reasoning and spiritual care, but include relevant and objective information that can help nurses in implementing spiritual care.

Interestingly, most clinical validation studies regarding the diagnoses related to spirituality have been conducted with adult patients (Chaves et al. 2010, Caldeira et al. 2016, 2017). Further clinical studies with children and adolescents are needed and nurses and midwives who work within these areas are crucial in this process. But, considering that nurses in the NICU care for parents and their family, some clinical indicators of spiritual distress may be adequate also in this context. Three major defining characteristics have been identified as relevant when patients are in spiritual distress: expressing suffering, lack of meaning in life and hopelessness (Chaves et al. 2010, Caldeira et al. 2016, 2017). When nurses are confronted with spiritual distress or grieving they should deliver the best support to the parents. Staff on a neonatal unit need to help in the journey of living with suffering in a transformative manner and as death approaches help parents find meaning and a way to move forward in life.

Nursing interventions, as said earlier, make sense if connected to a multidisciplinary approach, otherwise they could be empty of significance and effectiveness. Nurses need to be aware that providing spiritual care necessitates keeping parents and the babies central to any approaches to care delivery. The most effective spiritual care is that which targets parents' needs. So, the main intervention is presence and listening to parents requests. A comforting environment promotes security and trust in parents so that they do not feel abandoned. Within the hospital, nurses need to promote individualised care, creating an environment that will be familiar to parents. NICU's often allow and request parents to bring baby's clothes and objects. The baby is referred to by their name and this dignifies and celebrates life, regardless of the baby's health status. Parents who are religious may ask to pray or request the chaplain or spiritual leader visit. Praying is perceived as promoting a sense of wellbeing by mothers. Other interventions, listed in the Nursing Interventions Classifications, include listening, spiritual support and therapeutic touch (Bulechek et al. 2013).

This therapeutic touch relates to the nurse–patient relationship, but particularly in NICU, where parents can participate in therapeutic touch in parent-baby touching. Yet this is often difficult to perform due to the baby being in an incubator. Therefore all strategies that allow this touch need to be developed so that parents can provide care for their baby, e.g. feeding, clothing, encouraging skin-to-skin or kangaroo care. These moments of 'touch' can be moving for NICU staff and parents. The occasion of touch is concerned with sharing our humanity. Nurses providing spiritual care recognise the human nature of suffering and are able to feel empathy and compassion in a way that professional and clinical tasks are not disturbed.

When parents are suffering from spiritual distress the behaviour is similar to grieving (Dyer 2005). A model of 'three Ds' has been suggested to help nurses and NICU professionals in providing care: Derealisation, Denial and Dissociation (Dyer 2005). 'Derealisation' relates to supporting parents to keep functioning in hospital whilst away from the familiarity of home. 'Denial' occurs when parents and family are unwilling to accept and understand what has happened and 'Dissociation' is then that they are unable to effectively listen and understand the information given to them by NICU staff. The emotional, social and spiritual responses to these concerns are a way of addressing holistic care and adopting a multidimensional approach. Nurses and NICU professionals may find it difficult to start a conversation with grieving parents, but some verbal expressions and communication strategies have been suggested:

> I'm sad for you.
> How are you doing/coping with all of this?
> I don't know why it happened.
> What can I do for you?
> How can I help?
> What has been the hardest part for you?
>
> *(Dyer 2005, 28)*

These questions and statements favour empathy and the sense of being understood. Parents need to feel that this is a 'normal' journey they have to go through. With time and with the support they need, whether professional, groups of parents living similar experiences or family, they will continue to live their lives. Parents usually look for other parents on the Internet or through associations in order to connect with and provide support to each other. NICU professionals could provide this helpful information. Parents need to be advised to share their experiences with someone they trust; equally they should not feel pressured to do so if they do not wish to. The multidisciplinary approach should also include resources beyond the hospital: parishes, schools (in case they have other children) and in community healthcare services. The period in hospital could be the only time parents have with their baby, and nurses can promote strategies to ensure memories such as photos, a diary, the first clothes, the first feeding moment, the siblings' visit, the grandparents' visit, or others, that compose a 'memory record' of their unwell newborn who died.

The grieving journey hopefully ends in the acceptance stage, but this does not mean that parents would not suffer every time they remember the baby. That is why NICU professionals could keep contact with the parents for some days after the loss, making a call, sending a postcard or a letter. Parents will feel supported and feel valued and also feel that their baby had a dignified and valuable life that is remembered.

Appropriate training is needed regarding spirituality and spiritual care in the context of NICU when there is an unwell newborn who may die. The published literature highlights a need for training regarding NICU end of life care (Holms, Milligan and Kydd 2014, Cox and Wainwright 2015). Appropriate training could improve communication competencies and facilitate more 'sensitive communication' (Longmore 2016). Spiritual care in NICU requires further research so that more evidence informs practice, health policies and guidelines.

Conclusion

A child should represent the joy and meaning making of a new life. Sometimes the child is born earlier or unwell, and parents may be driven into a suffering situation and the loss of a child, widely known as the worst pain. Providing a holistic perspective of care needs to include recognition of the spiritual needs of parents and the spiritual approach to the care of the unwell newborn. Spiritual care is based on the therapeutic use of self and communication skills in promoting a spiritual environment where parents feel they can express beliefs and witness dignity-preserving care of their baby. Parents of an unwell baby are in a grieving process, and nurses and other NICU staff should assess, diagnose and perform the most effective interventions within a multidisciplinary approach. This approach needs to be maintained after the loss of a baby. A family needs to be provided with sensitive human support at this time so they can find meaning in life and ways of promoting spiritual wellbeing so that they can journey through this challenging time and continue with their lives.

Note

Figures 11.1, 11.2 and 11.3 in this chapter are original and created by the author.

References

Almeida, F., Moraes, M. and Cunha, M. 2016. "Taking Care of the Newborn Dying and their Families: Nurses' Experiences of Neonatal Intensive Care". *Journal of School of Nursing University of São Paulo* 50: 122–129. doi: http://dx.doi.org/10.1590/S0080-623420160000300018.

Attard, J., Baldacchino, D.R. and Camilleri, L. 2014. "Nurses' and Midwives' Acquisition of Competency in Spiritual Care: A Focus on Education". *Nurse Education Today* 34(12): 1460–1466. doi: 10.1016/j.nedt.2014.04.015.

Baldacchino D. 2006. "Nursing Competencies for Spiritual Care". *Journal of Clinical Nursing* 15(7): 885–896. doi: 10.1111/j.1365-2702.2006.01643.x.

Baldacchino, D. and Draper, P. 2001. "Spiritual Coping Strategies: A Review of the Nursing Research Literature". *Journal of Advanced Nursing* 34(6): 833–841.

Bélanger-Lévesque, M.N., Dumas, M., Blouin, S. and Pasquier, J.C. 2016. "'That was intense': Spirituality During Childbirth: A Mixed Method Comparative Study of Mothers' and Fathers' Experiences in a Public Hospital". *BMC Pregnancy and Childbirth* 16: 294. doi: 10.1186/s12884-016-1072-z.

Blencowe, H., Cousens, S., Chou, D., Oestergaard, M., Say, L., Moller, A.B., Kinney, M. and Lawn, J. 2013. "Born Too Soon: The Global Epidemiology of 15 Million Preterm Births". *Reproductive Health* 10 (Suppl 1): S2. doi: 10.1186/1742-4755-10-S1-S2.

Boss, R. and Clarke-Pounder, J. 2012. "Perinatal and Neonatal Palliative Care: Targeting the Underserved". *Progress in Palliative Care* 20(6): 343–348. doi: 10.1179/1743291X12Y.0000000039.

Bulechek, G.M., Butcher, H.K., Dochterman, J.M. and Wagner, C. 2013. *Nursing Interventions Classification (NIC)*. Philadelphia, PA: Elsevier.

Büssing, A., Föller-Mancini, A., Gidley, J. and Heusser, P. 2010. "Aspects of Spirituality in Adolescents". *International Journal of Children's Spirituality* 15: 25–44. doi: 10.1080/13644360903565524.

Caldeira, S., Carvalho, E.C. and Vieira, M. 2013. "Spiritual Distress – Proposing a New Definition and Defining Characteristics". *International Journal of Nursing Knowledge* 24(2): 77–84. doi: 10.1111/j.2047-3095.2013.01234.x.

Caldeira, S. and Hall, J. 2012. "Spiritual Leadership and Spiritual Care in Neonatology". *Journal of Nursing Management* 20(8): 1069–1075. doi: 10.1111/jonm.12034.

Caldeira, S. and Timmins, F. 2015. "Time as Presence and Opportunity: The Key to Spiritual Care in Contemporary Nursing Practice". *Journal of Clinical Nursing* 24(17–18): 2355–2356. doi: 10.1111/jocn.12909.

Caldeira, S., Timmins, F., Carvalho, E. and Vieira, M. 2016. "Nursing Diagnosis of 'Spiritual Distress' in Women with Breast Cancer". *Cancer Nursing* 39(4): 321–327. doi: 10.1097/NCC.0000000000000310.

Caldeira, S., Timmins, F., Carvalho, E. and Vieira, M. 2017. "Clinical Validation of the Nursing Diagnosis Spiritual Distress in Cancer Patients Undergoing Chemotherapy". *International Journal of Nursing Knowledge* 28(1): 44–52. doi: 10.1111/2047-3095.12105.

Callister, L.C. and Khalaf, I. 2010. "Spirituality in Childbearing Women". *Journal of Perinatal Education* 19(2): 16–24. doi: 10.1624/105812410X495514.

Cavaliere, T.A., Daly, B., Dowling, D. and Montgomery, K. 2010. "Moral Distress in Neonatal Intensive Care Unit RNs". *Advances in Neonatal Care* 10(3): 145–156. 10.1097/ANC.0b013e3181dd6c48.

Chaves, E., Carvalho, E.C., Souza, F. and Souza, L. 2010. "Clinical Validation of Impaired Spirituality in Patients with Chronic Renal Disease". *Revista Latino Americana de Enfermagem* 18(3): 309–316. doi: 10.1590/S0104-11692010000300003.

Christiansen, A., O'Brien, M., Kirton, J., Zubairu, K. and Bray, L. 2015. "Delivering Compassionate Care: the Enablers and Barriers". *British Journal of Nursing* 24(16): 833–837. doi: 10.12968/bjon.2015.24.16.833.

Cox, A. and Wainwright, L. 2015. "The Experience of Parents who Lose a Baby of a Multiple Birth During the Neonatal Period – a Literature Review". *Journal of Neonatal Nursing* 21(3): 104–113. doi: 10.1016/j.jnn.2014.11.003.

Crowther, S. and Hall, J. 2015. "Spirituality and Spiritual Care in and Around Childbirth". *Women and Birth* 28(2): 173–178. doi: 10.1016/j.wombi.2015.01.001.

Dyer, K. 2005. "Identifying, Understanding, and Working with Grieving Parents in the NICU, Part I: Identifying and Understanding Loss and the Grief Response". *Neonatal Network* 24(4): 35–46. doi: 10.1891/0730-0832.24.4.27.

Fosareli, P. 2012. "Care for Children". In *Oxford Textbook of Spirituality in Healthcare*, edited by M. Cobb, C. Puchalski and B. Rumbold, 243–249. New York: Oxford University Press.

Gale, G., Franck, L.S., Kools, S. and Lynch, M. 2004. "Parents' Perceptions of their Infant's Pain Experience in the NICU". *International Journal of Nursing Studies* 41(1): 51–58.

Giske, T. and Cone, P. 2015. "Discerning the Healing Path – How Nurses Assist Patient Spirituality in Diverse Health Care Settings". *Journal of Clinical Nursing* 24(19–20): 2926–2935. doi: 10.1111/jocn.12907.

Green, J., Darbyshire, P., Adams, A. and Jackson, D. 2016. "Nenonatal Nurses' Response to a Hypothetical Premature Birth Situation: What if it was my Baby?" *Nursing Ethics*. Advance online publication. doi: 10.1177/0969733016677871.

Herdman, H. and Kamitsuru, S. 2014. *Nursing Diagnoses – Definitions and Classification 2015–2017*. Oxford: Wiley Blackwell.

Holms, N., Milligan, S. and Kydd, A. 2014. "A Study of the Lived Experiences of Registered Nurses who have Provided End-of-life Care within an Intensive Care Unit". *International Journal of Palliative Nursing* 20(11): 549–556. doi: 10.12968/ijpn.2014.20.11.549.

Hwang, H.S., Kim, H.S., Yoo, I.Y. and Shin, H.S. 2013. "Parenting Stress in Mothers of Premature Infants". *Child Health Nursing Research* 19(1): 39–48. doi: 10.4094/chnr.2013.19.1.39.

International Council of Nurses. ICN Code of Ethics (2012). Accessed September 12 2016: www.icn.ch/images/stories/documents/about/icncode_english.pdf.

Kain, V.J. 2007. "Moral Distress and Providing Care to Dying Babies in Neonatal Nursing". *International Journal of Palliative Nursing* 13(5): 243–248. doi: 10.12968/ijpn.2007.13.5.23495.

Kain, V. 2011. "Exploring the Barriers to Palliative Care Practice in Neonatal Nursing: A Focus Group Study". *Neonatal, Paediatric and Child Health Nursing* 14(1): 9–14.

Longmore, M. 2016. "Neonatal Nursing: Palliative Care Guidelines". *Kai Tiaki Nursing New Zealand* 22(4): 36.

Mancini, A., Uthaya, S., Beardsley, C., Wood, D. and Modi, N. 2014. "Practical Guidance for the Management of Palliative Care on Neonatal Units". Accessed 20 September 2016 at www.uk-sands.org/sites/default/files/NICU-Palliative-Care-Feb-2014.pdf.

McSherry, W. 2006. "The Principal Components Model: A Model for Advancing Spirituality and Spiritual Care within Nursing and Health Care Practice". *Journal of Clinical Nursing* 15(7): 905–917. doi: 10.1111/j.1365-2702.2006.01648.x.

McSherry, W. and Smith, J. 2012. "Spiritual Care". In *Care in Nursing – Principles, Values and Skills*, edited by W. McSherry, R. McSherry and R. Watson, 117–131. New York: Oxford University Press.

Nascimento, L., Alvarenga, W., Caldeira, S., Mica, T., Oliveira, F., Pan, R., Santos, T., Carvalho, E.C. and Vieira, M. 2016. "Spiritual Care: The Nurses' Experiences in the Pediatric Intensive Care Unit". *Religions* 7: 27. doi:10.3390/rel7030027.

Nuzum, D., Meaney, S. and O'Donoghue, K. 2014. "The Impact of Stillbirth on Consultant Obstetrician Gynaecologists: a Qualitative Study". *British Journal of Obstetrics and Gynaecology* 121(8): 1020–1028. doi: 10.1111/1471-0528.12695.

Nuzum, D., Meaney, S. and O'Donoghue, K. 2016. "The Place of Faith for Consultant Obstetricians Following Stillbirth: A Qualitative Exploratory Study". *Journal of Religions and Health* 55(5): 1519–1528. doi: 10.1007/s10943-015-0077-7.

Prinds, C., Hvidt, N.C., Mogensen, O. and Buus, N. 2013. "Making Existential Meaning in Transition to Motherhood – A Scoping Review". *Midwifery* 30(6): 733–741. doi: 10.1016/j.midw.2013.06.021.

Ramezani, M., Ahmadi, F., Mohammadi, E. and Kazemnejad A. 2014. "Spiritual Care in Nursing: A Concept Analysis". *International Nursing Review* 61(2): 211–219. doi: 10.1111/inr.12099.

Reed, P., Smith, P., Fletcher, M. and Bradding, A. 2003. "Promoting the Dignity of the Child in Hospital". *Nursing Ethics* 10(1): 67–76.

Ribeiro, C., Moura, C., Sequeira, C., Barbieri, M. and Erdmann, A. 2015. "Parents' and Nurses' Perceptions of Nursing Care in Neonatology – An Integrative Review". *Referência* 4: 137–146. doi: 10.12707/RIV14023.

Rumbold, B. 2012. "Models for Spiritual Care". In *Oxford Textbook of Spirituality in Healthcare*, edited by M. Cobb, C. Puchalski and B. Rumbold, 177–183. New York: Oxford University Press.

Schroeder, J. 2008. "Ethical Issues for Parents of Extremely Premature Infants". *Journal of Paediatrics and Child Health* 44(5): 302–304. doi: 10.1111/j.1440-1754.2008.01301.x.

Section on Hospice and Palliative Medicine and Committee on Hospital Care. 2013. "Pediatric Palliative Care and Hospice Care Commitments, Guidelines, and Recommendations". *Pediatrics* 132(5): 966–972. doi:10.1542/peds.2013-2731.

Smith J. and McSherry, W. 2004. "Spirituality and Child Development: A Concept Analysis". *Journal of Advanced Nursing* 45(3): 307–315.

Soares, R., Christoffel, M., Rodrigues, E., Machado, E. and Cunha, A. 2016. "The Meanings of Caring for Pre-term Children in the Vision of Male Parents". *Texto e Contexto Enfermagem* 25(4): e1680015. doi: 10.1590/0104-07072016001680015.

Taylor, E. J., Petersen, C., Oyedele, O. and Haase, J. 2015. "Spirituality and Spiritual Care of Adolescents and Young Adults with Cancer". *Seminars in Oncology Nursing* 31(3): 227–241. doi: 10.1016/j.soncn.2015.06.002.

Van Leeuwen, R. and Cusveller, B. 2004. "Nursing Competencies for Spiritual Care". *Journal of Advanced Nursing* 48(3): 234–246. doi: 10.1111/j.1365-2648.2004.03192.x.

Weathers, E., McCarthy, G. and Coffey, A. 2016. "Concept Analysis of Spirituality: An Evolutionary Approach". *Nursing Forum* 51(2): 79–96. doi: 10.1111/nuf.12128.

World Health Organization (2012). "Born Too Soon – the Global Action Report on Preterm Birth". Accessed 12 September 2016: www.who.int/pmnch/media/news/2012/preterm_birth_report/en/.

12

PARENTHOOD AND SPIRITUALITY

José Miguel de Angulo and Luz Stella Losada

Introduction

The presence of an arriving infant can captivate or enchant all those present. Being captivated by this presence produces tremendous courage, especially in the mother so she can provide her infant with the best help. Greenberg and Morris (1974) describe how witnessing and connecting with this experience unleashes our capacity to feel connected with others and establishes secure emotional attachments with others closely connected with our lives. To witness birth is thus to have direct contact with our historical roots and our deep need to connect. The acknowledgment of the infant as a psychological, mental, volitional and spiritual being not only opens an incredible new world for the development of an infant but also gives parents access to a new world; a world in which they can have one of the most profound experiences a human being can have. To be present at birth is to be met by a unique opportunity for realigning the life trajectory of a new human being, their parents and other adults who may be present.

We ourselves are parents to five children who were born in very peaceful and familiar settings which allowed us to experience a profound bonding with each one of our children. Although we are Christians and our understanding of spirituality and birth is informed by our theological beliefs we also acknowledge that spirituality is always more than any one religion or belief system. We contend that childbirth is a universal human experience and from our personal and professional experiences there is no other time or place in our lives in which there is so much spiritual energy and fascination than at the miracle of emerging life. We begin with an infant's birth who we name Sonia.

Once upon a time there was the miracle of emerging life. Sonia arrived to our world yet doesn't have a clue why she has been sent to this strange and scary place. She knows only her powerful drive for survival, a drive that propels her in the face of all obstacles. Her brain tells her, "You must breathe in this very strange place. Breathe!" And so she gasps for those first few breaths. Her eyes inquisitively track the chaotic movement of incomprehensible shapes; the dazzling lights that flood the space around her. Unknown noises pump into her ears and brain, making things more chaotic. Her skin is bombarded by contact with unknown objects. Having been cast into the depth of life, she suddenly experiences the strangeness of gravity and the pain of intrusive physical sensations of being roughly touched that pushes and pulls without reason or explanation; then suddenly she lands on something that is warm and comforting. Things quiet down and her breath becomes more peaceful. She begins to hear that familiar rhythmic pumping that has accompanied her since the beginning of her existence. In all the chaos of her new world, two unmistakable voices pierce the noise to draw her attention. The synchronised high and low pitches and familiar smells create a soft gentle song she already knows; in that moment she feels "I'm not alone". The comforting sounds of her parents encourage her. Little by little she gains control of her arm and leg muscles and begins to crawl along ever so gently along her mother's abdomen toward the source of that enchanting scent.

Gradually, within her blurry field of vision, her mother's breast emerges, and she bobs her head from right to left, up and down as she responds to a powerful primordial drive. Sonia's wiggling and crawling is not in vain; each movement brings her a few millimetres closer to the nipple. Before she reaches the nipple, she must make extra efforts to control her neck and heavy head in order to properly achieve that vital first latch. Finally she has grasped her mother's soft nipple and suckles for the first time. This oral tactile moment is a fundamental survival strategy; this is Sonia's source of physical and emotional nutrition. The challenging experience of crawling up her mother's body ends with a pleasurable experience of suckling for food and comfort that she will repeat many times in the coming days and months. Her mother's nipple and breast will allow Sonia to recognise the feel of her mother in her mouth and acts as a powerful means for bonding and attachment.

Sonia's first emotional relationship is thus formed through multiple magic mechanisms that will develop the most incredible characteristic of humans, the ability to experience profound intimacy with other human beings. The type and quality of bonding experiences the baby has in the beginning of her life will establish the direction of her life as well as her capacity to experience empathy toward other human beings through life. The initial moments of life establish a sense of belongingness and love that mirrors what she was receiving through the umbilical cord. The cutting of Sonia's umbilical cord, which maintained an intimate relationship with her mother for 9 months, marks the development of a new emotional cord and physical attachment to her mother's breast. The placenta and uterus that warmly held and sustained her existence, which were suddenly removed at birth, are replaced by the "social uterus".

The social uterus is the bond between parents and the newborn providing a sense of safety, care and love. It is an exceptional experience that reconnects with the life giving force of the uterus, a force, we argue, that has been made invisible over the last century. The uterus is not simply a place where life begins. It is not simply the centre of a woman's life and sexuality that forms a foetus. Rather, it is our first home that gently surrounds us all on the journey to join the great family of humanity. Leaving this home Sonia has arrived into a chaotic world but also an incredible place initiating exciting feelings and experiences as she experiences a rush of sights, sounds and smells. As Sonia's parents provide her a loving, sustaining environment, the world gradually comes into focus and becomes less chaotic. Through gentle interaction, Sonia will soon learn to recognise faces and voices, establish foundational imprints for enjoyable and meaningful learning about how to move, understand language and make sense of what is around her during the coming months. The encounter between Sonia and her parents in the first two to three hours of life (that we would define as sacred time) establishes foundations for encounters with others they will share throughout life. These encounters contribute to an all-encompassing exquisite 'romantic dance of tenderness' that builds a family's socio-emotional caring life together.

Has Sonia's story of emerging new life been threatened by our 21st-century world, a world that has reduced birth to organic and medical measurable components? Have scientific advances that focus only on the management of biomedical complications covered over something significant, therefore preventing parents experiencing the mystery of birth?

Precious vessels of grace

When we open our minds and hearts to the profound mystery of new human life, to the moment of birth, to the majesty and marvel of a birth, we can experience exactly when the Hebrews described an infant as a channel of spiritual meaning and strength. The ancient Hebrews proclaimed the marvels of their God's grace and strength:

> O Lord, our Lord,
> How excellent is thy name in all the earth!
> Who hast set thy glory above the heavens.
> Out of the mouth of babes and sucklings
> Hast thou ordained strength …
>
> *(Psalm 8:1–2; King James Version)*

In the New Testament Jesus adds,

> I thank thee, O Father, Lord of heaven and earth, because thou hast hid these things from the wise and prudent, and hast revealed them unto babes.
> *(Matthew 11:25)*

From these Christian teachings infants are thus understood as a great door to understanding of the profundity of our existence and how we relate with each other. That is why Jesus talks about the Upside Kingdom in which God's message needs to be understood not from the perspective of the wise, but from the perspective of the children.

> Let the little children come to me, and stop keeping them away. For the kingdom of heaven belongs to people like these.
>
> *(Matthew 19:14)*

The implication is that we should place immense value on the newborn and children if we want to understand what 'kingdom of heaven' Jesus was talking about.

Encounters with infants provide a unique opportunity to enter into a special spiritual experience. An infant represents a shared mystery and reflects God's image and likeness. The opportunity to experience intimacy with an infant is an opportunity to experience the encounter with a human being that carries all the potential to be fully human that has not yet been distorted by the multiple troubles and vicissitudes of society. The child's brain has an incredible inbuilt capacity not only to analyse and grasp what is going on around her, but also to connect and synchronise with adults in such a way that profoundly transforms the adult's brain. There is emergent evidence of this synchronistic connectivity.

Parenting interactions with the baby generates brain plasticity in those parents experiencing profound changes (Leuner, Glasper and Gould 2010). Infants' capacity for connectedness and communication reaches out for interaction through eye contact and eye movements, babbling, facial expressions and gestures (Glocker et al. 2009, Strathearn, Fonagy and Montague 2008). The eagerness of the adults to be open and engage with this communication will shape the quality of relationships that infants will develop throughout life. What happens in this initial interaction will continue during the first months of life, and this will shape how an infant will relate to others through life (Grossmann and Grossmann 2009, Graham 2017).

We also need to work toward ensuring that the childbirth experience becomes a profound spiritual experience; one that allows parents to see how transcendent human beings actually are, and that we are not just a bunch of organs and biological processes; not merely a mass of tissues with mechanical interactions between organs, bones and muscles or just biochemical processes. Through the experience of caring for infants, parents and other adults can enter into a complete new way of relating. This requires immersion in what we call the 'romantic dance of tenderness' with the infant. This dance allows us to experience the greatness of what humans are and help lead us into a new interconnected compassionate society and overcome our broken, disconnected, polarised and fragmented world.

Romantic dance of tenderness

A newborn baby, like Sonia, who has taken an active part in her birth process, wakes up for around two hours. This time allows for interaction with parents, others and the world. Depending on how parents welcome and offer a nurturing sustaining environment, the baby will be able to reorganise and achieve a return to equilibrium. After two to three hours trying to interact with parents and the world, an infant usually falls asleep again, being awake the following days for only short periods of lime (7% to 10% of the day). The *first awakening* is caused by the birth from the comfortable mother's womb, from a "resting" or sleeping state in utero, to a radical very different environment. This allows the infant to initiate the process of developing her capacity to take care of herself that is beautifully expressed through the crawling, pursuing her new source of nutrition on mother's breast (Gangal 2007). This is her first life project, proactively pursuing reconnection with the mother and looking for the nipple. Impairing this crawling and latching on to the nipple deprives all present in those moments of the magnificent display of energy and capacity of the baby caring for her own life. This situation is prevented if any other object other than the nipple is introduced because initial oral tactile imprinting is crucial. Any inanimate object such as a dummy or bottle feeding will disrupt this part of the dance after birth. The infant will displace her emotional oral tactile fixation onto the object, seriously obstructing the first latch and therefore the first emotional relationship that is formed through the infant's behaviour of suckling (Mobbs et al. 2016).

Other unconscious insensitive actions at birth may have a strong impact on infants. Frequently, powerful hands of adults display an intrusive and forceful action of grasping the baby and moving her without any sensitivity to her desires and capacities. This can occur at a time when procedures occur, such as weighing and measuring that are less important than the effort of the baby trying to gain equilibrium and reorganise herself through the bonding and interaction with her mother. The initial connections with her mother should not be undermined by such ill-timed, non-urgent clinical procedures. The mysterious experience of birth is beautifully enriched by the immersion in the romantic dance of tenderness between the infant and her mother as well as with all who have been invited to be there. Parents, and specially the father/partner, have an incredible window of opportunity to introduce themselves and welcome the infant into a caring and loving community, and to experience immersion in this romantic dance of tenderness.

The time after birth is crucial for many reasons: for breastfeeding success; building ongoing capacity to deal with stress and potential threats; and the establishment of foundational relationships. Relationships are part of our spiritual expression as shown throughout this book. Developing this capacity to establish secure attachments and relationships is important. Evidence has revealed how these relationships are central to an infant's cognitive development, a robust brain architecture and capacity to establish healthy relationships through life (Borra, Iacovou and Sevilla 2012, Sean et al. 2013). Denying the optimal opportunities for forming these foundational early relationships may have consequences on the spiritual wellbeing of the infant.

Becoming parents

The human infant is the most socially influenced creature on earth; the adult that interacts with an infant is undergoing the most influential experience s/he may have during her/his life. We contend that the way we initiate the first minutes of an infant's arrival strongly shapes the direction of how we are re-born as parents. Becoming parents opens a new horizon to see the world from a very different perspective, bringing forth new ways of feeling and learning that reorganise all our prior experiences and behaviours. It is like a second opportunity to be born, not as a baby but as a parent. These magical moments at birth can become the initiation of an adventure that allow transformation and tenderness. Yet this is not always the case in all newly forming families. Unfortunately, the traditional hierarchical parent–child relations, based on the "exercise of authority over the child", not only seriously erode the potential development of a child's ability to self-regulate and achieve self-agency, but parents too suffer the consequences and are left bereft of what could have been possible. Hierarchical parent–child relations can close possibilities for adults to enter an exciting world where their children generate profound transformational opportunities for parents. In this hierarchical worldview of parenting the parent's role is seen as responsible for influencing and moulding the child. Thus, open parenting does not seek to tame, control and socialise their infant: it yields to the possibilities brought by their infant as they as parents become touched and transformed. Open parenting develops an appreciation of how their infant will grow into a human being who is full of grace and beauty and who has come as a gift into their lives. When parents are open to that new horizon, a profound beautiful transformational awaits them.

Birth and society

Advances in neuroscience provide more evidence of the significance of relationality in and around birth. A French study describes the profound changes in the brain architecture of the mother as result of the interaction with the infant.

> Profound behavioural changes occur in the mother at parturition, together with extensive remodelling of neural circuits. These changes include neurochemical, morphological and functional plasticity. The continuous generation of new neurones in the hippocampus and the olfactory system is an additional form of neuroplasticity that contributes to motherhood. (…) Oestradiol, corticosterone and prolactin changes associated with

parturition are the main physiological factors involved in the regulation of neurogenesis that have been determined so far.

(Lévy, Gheusi and Keller 2011, 984)

Lévy et al.'s work has profound importance for society as a whole. Neuroscience is revealing for the first time how the delicate biological and physiological processes around birth are part of the mystery of emergent life. Sensitivity toward the foetus' development as a precious and desired human being can predict patterns of interactions after the baby's birth. Parents' sensitivity is linked to their ability to "mentalise" about their child, how to perceive, interpret and affectively share and mirror a young child's emotional states. This sensitivity leads to a high capacity for responding to infant distress (Flykt 2014, Rosenblum et al. 2008). Modifications of mental representations of unborn infants by pregnant women living in impoverished conditions affect the future of that mother, her mental health and the way she interacts with the infant. There is a lot of evidence now that supports the claim that this can in turn change the child's future (Arnott and Meins 2007, Alhusen et al. 2013, Nishikawa and Sakakibara 2013, Bellieni et al. 2007, Abasi et al. 2013). These studies show how it is possible to bring radical changes about in the life of future generations without necessarily waiting until social health determinants can be transformed. In other words how birth is experienced by the infant and parents potentially has major implications for society.

The World Health Organization published "Social determinants of health: The solid facts" (World Health Organization 2003). It stated that actions for health need to be geared towards addressing the social factors affecting wellbeing in order to attack the causes of ill health before they can lead to problems. It showed the strength of the scientific evidence on social determinants and presented them in a clear and understandable form. However, even though social health determinants strongly shape us from a very young age the type of person we will become is not necessarily due to these documented factors alone. We contend that it is possible to improve society's health and wellbeing by proactively optimising conditions that promote development of healthy infant brain architecture during the first days of life. In one of our previous published papers we show how neuroscience research reveals that being born human does not necessarily ensure an infant will become humane (de Angulo and Losada 2015). Rather, the ability to live harmoniously with other humans and with nature in a meaningful and healthy way are linked to the infant brain's capacity to understand others, to care, to share, to listen, to value and to be empathetic. The foundation of these characteristics is established in early infancy by the experience of being cared for, shared with, listened to, valued and nurtured. Humane caregiving fosters a brain architecture that is able to express our capacity to be humane. Inhumane caregiving erodes our human capacity to be humane. Our previous work has shown how families with high socioeconomic limitations can make a radical difference in the way their children relate, learn and thrive for life when parents learn through pregnancy how their baby is a psychological, mental and volitional agent that is eager to interact with them and to become a transforming force in that family and society (de Angulo and Losada 2015, 2016).

When parents open their minds to the amazing world of the infants' development, especially concerning interactions, they will appreciate how parenting behaviours directly influence their infants' brain. They will be able to develop the capacity to see, listen and interact in a very radical, different way with that infant from birth but also before the birth and intrauterine period. It has been demonstrated that maternal preconceptions about parenting are also considered predictors of a child's temperament, sensitivity and empathy with good pro-social behaviours, even for mothers belonging to low socioeconomic groups (Kiang, Moreno and Robinson 2004). Therefore, poverty alone is not necessarily the major cause of poor socioemotional development in infants. Secure attachment is a powerful force creating an "enduring affective tie" that has a "strong reciprocal" quality (parent-to-infant and infant-to-parent) that generates changes in all those involved (Condon, Corkindale and Boyce 2008). The power of brains to shape each other in paternal/maternal–foetus/infant interactions was unknown until this century. Therefore, how we engage with infants is even more crucial than we thought before.

Still, in western society there are many people who think that the magical moments of first interactions with an infant are something that has to do with what is called "maternal instinct". However, more evidence is emerging that reveals how fathers can also experience profound emotions on welcoming and caring for an infant. It appears that these paternal experiences also cause our brains to re-wire. It is now accepted that this plasticity is inherent in brain physiology and generates changes in neuron networks in response to external influences. Several studies show how the brain of the father alters when they actively engage in caring practices for their infant:

> Since there's no clear physical connection between a father and his child – at least not like the one seen with mom and baby – researchers are starting to look deep in the brain for better clues to understand the power of this relationship. A recent wave of studies are starting to bear fruit … We are now learning that in the first few days after birth, changes occur in the brains of both the dad and the baby, depending on whether the father is around or not. Perhaps neuroscientists have finally cornered the elusive father–child bond, and found the biological hook that makes sure a father sticks around after birth.
>
> *(Mossop 2010, 1)*

When fathers engaged in primary-caregiving, they exhibited high amygdala activation similar to mothers, alongside high superior temporal sulcus (STS) activation comparable to fathers, and functional connectivity between amygdala and STS. It was found that time spent by the father in childcare correlated with amygdala-STS connectivity. Findings describe mechanisms of brain malleability or plasticity with caregiving experiences in human fathers. This research showed how hands-on parenting reconfigures the brain of a father in the same way that pregnancy and childbirth reconfigures the mother's brain (Abrahama et al. 2014). It appears relationships can literally generate changes in the parents' brains, producing new way of thinking, behaviour and engaging with the world.

> The brains of parents are clearly different from those of non-parents, having been changed by the presence of offspring and corresponding hormonal fluctuations. Available evidence suggests that structural reorganization occurs in the hippocampus and PFC of mothers and fathers
>
> *(Leuner, Glasper and Gould 2010, 9)*

The potential for transformation during interaction between parents and infants has wider implications. Emergent relationships after birth, we would suggest, may have a strong societal significance.

Our discussion has shown how children, especially when they are infants, are the good news for the world. We would contend that it is imperative to change our mental representations of infants and see them as gifts and perhaps society's future salvation. Infants are valuable to us individually and to society; they bring a reflection of the divine into this world. Today, neuroscience is showing us that newborn brains are not empty and neither are they passive recipients of adults' educational activities. On the contrary, infants carry in their brains inbuilt principles about being human and a reflection of creation. An infant's brain has an incredible inbuilt capacity not only to analyse and grasp what is going on around them but an incredible capacity to connect with adults and produce profound transformations in the brains of the adults they interact with. This inbuilt capacity and quality for bonding and attachment is the fundamental glue for families, communities and society. Our survival as a species may be dependent on these early formative relationships. When an infant is able to live in constant proximity to her caregiver we are all changed. These relationships (or lack of them) may determine who we become as adults, how we interact with others and all of life, human and non-human. If we accept that our brains and our ability to feel love, trust, express affection and empathy or compassion is directly influenced by our relationships around birth, then we must collectively take responsibility.

The miracle of emerging life is sacred. The sacred moment of emergent life can be fully experienced when the dreams and aspirations of the women and couple are addressed. This requires the full agency of the mother in planning for the birth including making decisions about the place, the people she wants to have around and the type of support she would like to have. The health care system needs to play a new role, providing comprehensive support beyond the traditional reductionist, risk-management approach. The role of the partner cannot be just a support person but must be an active partner in the process. To be witness to the birth of a new human being and watch the unfolding of a new life into relationship with others is one of the most profound and spiritual experiences individuals can enjoy. To be part of and engage in the romantic dance of tenderness is to be immersed in a journey of spiritual transformation. The miracle of emerging life has a transformative energy that reminds us that a better world is always possible.

Health care systems and health research need to re-orientate. They need to focus on understanding what is going on in the brain during pregnancies and parenting. This in turn needs to inform our contemporary approaches to maternity care, moving us beyond purely bio-medical concerns. This requires a transdisciplinary team involving midwives, psychologies, educators and social workers, among others, to promote a holistic approach to the miracle of a woman giving birth to life, to another human being. To be witness to this miracle of life coming into being is to be rendered speechless. Many people say about birth 'I cannot describe with words what I have experienced ... after this experience I will never be the same.' It is obvious to us that it is time for a paradigm shift in maternity services and the way society speaks of childbirth.

Infants do not come as a "tabula rasa" (blank slate) that we need to mould. In the Christian tradition Jesus presented a radically different understanding of what humanity is.

> Truly I tell you, whoever doesn't receive the kingdom of God as a little child will never get into it at all.
>
> *(Luke 18:17)*

We would urge society to listen to our children. It is they who gift the transforming, healing force for our broken infancies and lead us into new ways of relating.

> The greatest lessons in life if we would but stoop and humble ourselves, we would learn not from grown-up learned men, but from the so-called ignorant children ... if we would approach babes in humility and in innocence, we would learn wisdom from them.
>
> *(Gandhi 1931)*

This may seem like an unreachable spiritual ideal. This is a call that challenges all parents, all who work in and around childbirth and society as a whole. A peaceful and harmonious civilisation for humankind will start when the wellbeing of the infant prevails over any other consideration. The overcoming of violence will start when infants experience peaceful births and loving families in the initial period of their lives. If we change the beginning, the whole story will be different for that child, her family and community.

If we hope to create a non-violent world where respect and kindness replace fear and hatred, we must begin with how we treat each other at the beginning of life. For that is where our deepest patterns are set. From these roots grow fear and alienation – or love and trust.

(Suzanne Arms quote cited in Peterson 2015, XV)

Are you willing to begin and contribute to a radical new way of seeing, listening and interacting with infants? Are you willing to be part of our world's spiritual reawakening and renaissance?

References

Abasi, E. et al. 2013. The effect of maternal–fetal attachment education on maternal mental health. *Turkish Journal of Medical Sciences*, 43(5): 815–828.

Abrahama, E. et al. 2014. Father's brain is sensitive to childcare experiences. *Proceedings of the National Academy of Science*, 111(27): 9792–9797.

Alhusen, J.L. et al. 2013. A longitudinal study of maternal attachment and infant developmental outcomes. *Arch Women's Mental Health*, 16(6): 521–529.

Arnott, B. and Meins, E. 2007. Links between antenatal attachment representations, postnatal mind-mindedness, and infant attachment security: A preliminary study of mothers and fathers. *Bulletin of the Menninger Clinic*, 71: 132–149.

Bellieni, C.V. et al. 2007. Is prenatal bonding enhanced by prenatal education courses? *Minerva Ginecologica*, 59(2): 125–129.

Borra, C., Iacovou, M. and Sevilla, A. 2012. The effect of breastfeeding on children's cognitive and noncognitive development. *Labour Economics*, 19(4): 496–515.

Condon, J.T., Corkindale, C.J. and Boyce, P. 2008. Assessment of postnatal paternal-infant attachment: development of a questionnaire instrument. *Journal of Reproductive and Infant Psychology*, 26(3): 195–210.

de Angulo, J.M. and Losada, L.S. 2015. Health paradigm shifts in the 20th century. *Christian Journal for Global Health*, 2(1): 49–58.

de Angulo, J.M. and Losada, L.S. 2016. The emerging health paradigm in the 21st century: The formative first 1000 days of life. *Christian Journal for Global Health*, 3(2): 113–128. doi: https://doi.org/10.15566/cjgh.v3i2.38.

Flykt, M. 2014. *Prenatal representations predicting parent–child relationship in transition to parenthood.* Tampere University Press. https://tampub.uta.fi/bitstream/handle/10024/95679/978-951-44-9503-8.pdf?sequence=1

Gandhi, M. 1931. Speech at the Montessori Training College, London published in the newspaper *Young India*, on 19 November 1931. http://www.peace.ca/montessoriandgandhi.htm

Gangal, P. 2007. Initiation of breastfeeding by Breast Crawl. UNICEF India.

Glocker, M.L. et al. 2009. Baby schema in infant faces induces cuteness perception and motivation for caretaking in adults. *Ethology*, 115: 257–263.

Graham, M. 2017. *Nurturing natures: Attachment and children's emotional, sociocultural and brain development.* Abingdon: Routledge.

Greenberg, M. and Morris N. 1974. Engrossment: The newborn's impact upon the father. *American Journal of Orthopsychiatry*, 44(4): 520–531.

Grossmann, K. and. Grossmann, K.E. 2009. The impact of attachment to mother and father and sensitive support of exploration at an early age on children's psychosocial development through young adulthood. *Encyclopedia on Early Childhood Development*, Montreal: CEED, pp. 6–12.

Kiang, L., Moreno, A.J. and Robinson, J.L. 2004. Maternal preconceptions about parenting predict child temperament, maternal sensitivity, and children's empathy. *Developmental Psychology*, 40(6): 1081–1092.

Leuner, B., Glasper, E.R. and Gould, E. 2010. Parenting and plasticity. *Trends in Neurosciences*, 33(10): 465–473. doi:10.1016/j.tins.2010.07.003.

Lévy, F., Gheusi, G. and Keller, M. 2011. Plasticity of the parental brain: A case for neurogenesis. *Journal of Neuroendocrinology*, 23(11): 984–993.

Mobbs, E.J., Mobbs, G.A. and Mobbs, A.E.D. 2016. Imprinting, latchment and displacement: A mini review of early instinctual behaviour in newborn infants influencing breastfeeding success. *Acta Pædiatrica*, 105: 24–30.

Mokhtar, M. 2007. Effects of attachment on early and later development. *The British Journal of Developmental Disabilities*, 53(105): 81–95.

Mossop, B. 2010. The brains of our fathers: Does parenting rewire dads? Fathers and their children reshape one another's neurons. *Scientific American*. 17 August 2010. www.scientificamerican.com/article/the-brains-of-our-fathers/

Nishikawa, M. and Sakakibara, H.E. 2013. Effect of nursing intervention program using abdominal palpation of Leopold's maneuvers on maternal-fetal attachment. *Reproductive Health*, 10: 12.

Peterson, C. 2015. *The mindful parent: Strategies from peaceful cultures to raise compassionate, Competent Kids*. New York: Skyhorse Publishing.

Rosenblum, K.L. et al. 2008. Reflection in thought and action: Maternal parenting reflectivity predicts mind-minded comments and interactive behavior. *Infant Mental Health Journal*, 29: 362–376.

Sean, C.L., Deoni, S.C.L. et al. 2013. Breastfeeding and early white matter development: A cross-sectional study. *NeuroImage*, 82: 77–86.

Strathearn, L., Li, J., Fonagy, P., and Montague, P.R. 2008. What's in a smile? Maternal brain responses to infant facial cues. *Pediatrics*, 122: 40–51.

World Health Organization. 2003. Social determinants of health: The solid facts. Copenhagen, Denmark: WHO. Available from: http://www.euro.who.int/__data/assets/pdf_file/0005/98438/e81384.pdf

PART III

Pulling the threads together

13

CONCLUSION

'There is something going on at birth!'

Jenny Hall and Susan Crowther

We are both 'crafters' – Jenny 'creates' for pleasure as well as for practicality; Susan, a crafter of stories from lived experience descriptions. It is therefore not by chance that we have included 'threads' in the title of this final chapter, as we are attempting to weave into a coherent whole the 'weft' that has been created by the different authors. The beautiful, inspirational colours they have created have melded together to provide a complex picture that underpins our statement that 'there is something going on at birth'.

Jenny has been contemplating the issues raised in this book for nearly 40 years of being around health care and midwifery in particular, and through personal experience of motherhood. Susan has been exploring what it means to live and experience spirituality in her personal and professional life having been transformed through the witnessing of numerous births as a midwife. The understanding of humanity as 'not just physical beings', and the privilege of being present at the end of life and at the beginnings, has inspired us to discuss, debate and write across continents and at last, return together in the birthing of this project. It has been heartening over time to recognise that we are not alone in our musings; there are many (if not all?) present at births all over the world who stand in awe at the wonder of creation, often feeling overwhelmed at the dawn of each new life. It remains a mystery (though many are still trying to understand the science of it all) how a couple of cells join together to become a human baby, and subsequently create a mother and a new family.

We have been wondering though if this element of mystery has become hidden away and avoided in the current contexts of maternity care in developed nations, where the language of 'risk' and 'safety' have become prevalent among the voices of medicalisation in what is inherently a 'non-medical', 'natural' process. Those present at birth are perhaps more afraid to talk about the powerful meanings of pregnancy and birth through fear of ridicule or fear this is not 'evidence-based'. There is, however, significant experiential evidence within the chapters of this book. Each chapter is brimming with stories from women and their carers gesturing to something more about childbirth than a purely medicalised, tick-box process. This book highlights that there is indeed 'something going on at birth' beyond the everyday focus on risk, safety and medical language.

Reflecting on the content

As we indicated in the introduction we have come from a philosophical stance that pregnancy-birth-postnatal are one continual process; we challenge the demarcation between these 'parts' of childbirth and prefer to view the childbirth year as an integrated whole. It is therefore no surprise to us that our chapter authors, although charged with writing about specific aspects of this continuum, remained holistically focused and continually strayed into other 'parts' of the childbirth year.

As you read through the chapters of this book questions about your own philosophy and approaches to pregnancy and birth may have arisen. Indeed the content may have started you on a different path of thinking and feeling about childbirth. Each chapter invites us into new horizons of understanding; at the same time, the book as a whole gifts a depth of knowing and hopefully leaves you with an opportunity to pause and reflect. The implications of each individual chapter's contents and all chapters together could have far-reaching consequences if we were all to ponder the messages more carefully.

We acknowledge that there is always more to say about this phenomenon. One book would never be able to cover all perspectives. Much remains unsaid, other religious, cultural and ethnic groups and practices could have been incorporated. We also acknowledge that not all topics touching childbirth and spirituality have been included – for example, infertility, surrogacy, adoption, lone and same sex parenting. Our intention has been to expose new horizons of understanding and begin a dialogue. Although we have provided some breadth of perspectives our focus has been on depth rather than lightly covering all topics.

Birth as sacred and holy

Within these chapters the notion of birth as a sacred or holy event to be respected and revered is commented upon regularly. Within her chapter 'Childbirth as a sacred celebration' (Chapter 2) Susan refers to the special 'felt-time' at birth as 'Kairos time', a deeply meaningful place where life is changed at that moment for everyone present. But it is also the place where there is an intergenerational 'shift' that brings connectedness into the past as well as the potential this new life brings to the future of that family and society. In Kairos time we are addressed by our shared natality. In Carolyn's and Céline's chapter, 'Holding sacred space in labour and birth' (Chapter 7), they highlight that birth is a place of mystery and call for a 're-enchantment' of birth, and to honour it. These two chapters indicate that something has been 'lost' and needs to be 'found' again within our current birth practices.

The past and present are also explored by Anna's visual chapter, 'Ritual and Art in a Philosophy of Birth' (Chapter 3), as she unpacks the artworks created depicting birth across the centuries. Anna presents artworks and draws attention to the sacredness of certain images and how they connect women across countries and continents as symbols of something Earthly yet divine. She also addresses the value of art as a tool to 'sacralise' pregnancy and birth. However, we also need to acknowledge that what was valued in the past needs to be balanced with the reality that historical birth practices and some traditional birth practices were not always 'safe'. None of the chapter authors deny that contemporary medical learning has, in many cases, saved lives; what we contend is that spirituality in and around childbirth needs our collective consideration. As discussed by Carolyn and Céline, the spiritual aspects of life are not 'add-ons'; they are aspects of being human and are part of all life and therefore inherent to a woman's experience in whatever situation.

Jenny's (H) chapter, 'Pregnancy and the unborn child' (Chapter 4) brings the focus closely to the unborn baby. Jenny shows us that pregnancy is 'sacred' as it is carrying another human being who is body-mind-spirit. She describes how the complexity of this situation is recognised through seeing how deeply the mother and baby are entwined; two people as one. Jenny discusses how this involvedness is enhanced in the social context of the mother and family, as cultural philosophies impact on the views and values of the woman toward her unborn. She concludes that we need to consider how to enhance this sacred relationship as it is an important step in promoting spiritual wellbeing of both a woman and her baby.

In Jenny Parratt's chapter, 'Couple's spiritual experiences at birth' (Chapter 8) the focus turns to labour and the spiritual concept of women 'being in the moment', and of shifting into moments of the 'non-rational' with a 'deeply altered non-ordinary conscious state'. The women in Jenny's study are able to describe choices of deeply 'feeling' the sensations within their bodies and ascribing spiritual embodied meaning. Birth as sacred and holy weaves throughout the chapters attuning us into a deeper spiritual awareness about childbirth.

Childbirth as transitioning and transforming

As we saw in Chapters 1 and 2 the notion of transformation is central to many interpretations of spirituality. Therefore it is unsurprising that experiences of transformation emerge frequently throughout all the chapters. This is particularly apparent in Ingela's chapter, 'Spiritual questions during childbearing' (Chapter 5). Ingela shows how women face and meet the unknown as they transition from pregnancy to birth. She reveals through experiential stories how pregnancy itself is a place of transformation, where women focus on the past, present and future at different stages. Ingela describes this as a 'border' space – a space that is an existential place of meaning. She suggests that it is a place where women may 'develop strength and suffering'. The transitional space Ingela presents is akin to the temporal space named 'Kairos time' in Susan's chapter (Chapter 2). In that mysterious time-space the baby becomes a tangible person, where before they have been hidden from view. This is a time like no other, Susan suggests, bringing proximity to the feeling of sacredness when seen and unseen touch, when others far, near, physical and non-physical converge, when the significance, meaningfulness and purpose of human life becomes magnified.

A dance of spaces, places and relationships

Within the place of birth the midwife, partner and other health carers also have a spiritually significant and meaningful role. Ingela (Chapter 5) describes how a woman will be cared for by a midwife who is present in stillness, 'anchored' and solid. Such a midwife believes in the woman she cares for, recognising her limits while recognising the limits of her own professional behaviour too. Ingela proffers the image of an anchor in the storm – a place of solid safety and security. In Carolyn and Céline's chapter (Chapter 7) this quality is named 'holding the space'. As such, a midwife holds sacred space for the woman and baby where they can meet each other in wholeness. The midwife has a responsibility to 'hold the space' in Carolyn and Céline's chapter, and in Jenny's (P) chapter (Chapter 8) those with a labouring woman are to be 'guardians' of the birth space and 'hold the space' for a woman to 'own' her birth. In these chapters the midwife has a philosophy of openness to potential of meaning. The midwife is described as the 'greater than that' and referred to as the guardian of the 'passages'.

Jenny (P) highlights how the midwife needs to provide a 'safe' environment and for the woman to have complete trust. Within this space, too, the woman's partner is enabled to be a participant and a support. They, too, will experience the powerful, meaningful, spiritual nature of birth. The midwife, therefore, has the power to create this space of holiness, in the environment, and also the power to prevent it. The midwife as spiritual 'guardian' is exhorted to 'be' more rather than 'do' more (Carolyn and Céline) and to 'being there' (Jenny P). The onus, therefore, is on the midwife and how she has awareness of the space and herself. As Ingela shows us, the physical environment where birth takes place needs to bring calm and safety. Ingela contends that birth unfolds in a special place where a woman needs to be able to 'own' the room. One needs to question if these insights to ways of being in and around childbirth are possible in our contemporary maternity institutions and current models of care.

For Alison in her chapter, 'Spiritual obstetrics' (Chapter 9) the onus also lies with the medical team. Her exploration of the effect of attempting to control the birth space by medicine exposes how such controlling influences transform birth environments. Alison argues for a change of behaviours that are more attuned to holistic awareness and openness to more than the biomedical understandings. She tells us that doctors, too, may experience the sacred in the birth experience. Why would they not? However, there are many who would deny, turn away or avoid such interpretations of childbirth. Her suggestion that some doctors 'apply love the wrong way' is profound. Alison's message to all who provide maternity care is to be sensitive, receptive and enabling. Opening all our eyes to view the world in a different way of loving would transform childbirth in the 21st century.

Transforming broken futures

Not all childbirth experiences are optimal, not all women, infants and families traverse the childbirth year without concerns. Childbirth for some women and families may be a time of trauma and suffering as they come to terms with what may be broken future possibilities. The carer's role is key to alleviating their fears and anxieties. Three chapters explore traumatic and difficult situations that can arise in the childbirth year from several perspectives. What these chapters reveal is that far from being 'unspiritual and un-sacred or less significant' they are often experienced as an opportunity for spiritual growth. Gill's chapter, 'Growth and renewal through traumatic birth' (Chapter 10) highlights, through provocative narrative examples, of how stressful and traumatic childbirth events can offer women new possibilities and meanings through post-traumatic growth. Gill's work shows us how women facing the need to 'overcome' difficult circumstances may be enabled to find meaning and new life purpose, improved meaningful relationships, deeper spiritual understandings and self-growth. Gill's chapter challenges current discourses about how certain types of birth that are distressing and stressful experiences are not devoid of spiritual growth. Spiritual growth, Gill asserts, is not exclusive to a normal physiological birth. She argues for a more salutogenic perspective of childbirth, a perspective on wellness and spirituality and not biomedical pathology.

In Sílvia's chapter 'Spirituality when a newborn is unwell' (Chapter 11), we are confronted with the undesirable dilemma of when an infant is sick. Sílvia's work brings light to the changing family dynamics and internal questioning about the meaning of such circumstances related to individual existence and life. The heart-wrenching challenges are evocatively presented as those affected are faced with opportunities to reflect on their own identity, life journey and the meaning of their existence when living through such difficult times. As with Gill's chapter, challenging circumstances are understood as catalysts for spiritual growth. This spiritual growth includes meaning seeking, keeping hope and holding beliefs that may or may not be connected to religiosity; vis-à-vis religion is not a prerequisite for spiritual experience and spiritual growth.

Sílvia's work highlights the importance of nurses and midwives providing contextualised human and professional care when perinatal outcomes are uncertain and the possibility of an infant dying is real. Although care in these situations must include technical skills in a multidisciplinary health care team, the main quality required, Sílvia contends, is communication and relationship skills, including expression of empathy, compassion and awareness about the spiritual dimensions of life. In Joan's chapter 'Pregnancy loss and complexity' (Chapter 6), relationships are central and we are moved by descriptions of the complex personal adjustment to hope and meaning required when there is a diagnosis of a child's abnormality. Joan clearly illustrates how the context of their society and the religious underpinnings impacts on the difficult decisions women choose. How health professionals interact with women and their families in these challenging and distressing times is decisive in what will unfold. It is evident that the relationships health carers develop with women and families is key to enhancing hope and acceptance when things go wrong and when outcomes are not as expected. Families need to transform their broken futures into opportunities for spiritual growth. For this to be facilitated relationships are crucial. Relationships can help women and families integrate their experiences through meaning making and finding a sense of purpose as they move forward in their lives.

Power of relationships

What becomes increasingly evident in these chapters is the significance of relationships and sanctity of an opening felt-space in physical places that needs safeguarding. Even in hospital environments childbirth's potency shifts the mood of places, and those working in and around childbirth need to attune to one another in a specific way that engenders connection and wholeness. The power of relationships is highlighted throughout and culminates in José and Luz Stella's evocative chapter 'Parenthood and spirituality' (Chapter 12). In this final chapter we are addressed by the meaningful and significant spiritual nature of the parenting relationship. Although the chapter is largely informed by Christian theology, it reveals a significance in the early parenting relationships that extend beyond religious differences, the time of birth and the birthing room to the wider family, community and society as a whole. José and Luz Stella draw our awareness to the ever-unfolding evidence from multiple disciplines, including neurobiology studies. They reveal how these early human relationships are not only providing the necessary attachment required for an infant to thrive but have profound consequences on our entire lives as we build relationships throughout our lifetime. Their chapter brings us back to the notion of transformation at individual and societal level. They leave us pondering what we must do, inviting us to take action for the future of human society. If spirituality is defined in simple terms as an experience comprised of several recurring qualities, namely, transformational, relational, meaning-giving and sense of purpose, then the chapters of this book individually and collectively illustrate how childbirth is spiritual through and through.

What have we learned for the future?

In devising and editing this book one hope we have is that it will inspire some to action, to attune to spirituality in ways not previously articulated in such depth. We hope to have inspired more debate and discussion, as well as a decision to consider wider creation of evidence. However, we have not intended to present a view that totally opposes the present biomedical approach and create a false dichotomy with holistic spiritual care. This, we believe, is not a useful stance to take, and one that may cause division. Instead, we recognise that birth is a powerful, meaningful spiritual event, whether it is straightforward or complicated, and that the woman-baby-family deserve for their spiritual selves to be acknowledged and respected during all care encounters. No birthing story is more or less spiritual than others, and women's stories, alongside those of her partner, families, midwives and other health care providers should be honoured. There is no doubt that holistic approaches to care that include spirituality of childbirth are more than the current models and systems of care and discourses. Instead, spirituality and childbirth includes all types of births, all places of birth and includes everyone, whatever professional or non-professional group, those far and near, seen and unseen, those privileged to be in the room where birth happens and to all those in our society. Even if you have never been at a birth you cannot fail to be touched by birth's specialness and message of hope.

The voices and stories in this book bring a changing story of childbirth that attunes to spiritual meanings. They also lead to different ways of practice that are sensitive, compassionate and respectful of humanity, that bring a deeper connectedness which transcends any differences. What if this could be the 'truth' for every encounter in pregnancy and birth, where the richness of relationships is the key tool for care? There is enough evidence that points to the importance of meaningful social support during pregnancy and during birth. Building relationships that are life-affirming and recognising the woman as a person in her own right is spiritually affirming.

What if we recognised every pregnancy as significant? What if we were to encourage women during the pregnancy to focus and engage only on positive images of birth and beyond? Would this be a step towards reducing anxiety and fear and dispel some of the myths that are presented through current televised stories? For many years, women have been encouraged to visualise the space where they would give birth as a safe space and to undertake birth art for therapeutic reasons and to make meaning. The current craze of using colouring books as a way to calm and address mental health needs has branched out into pregnancy and may be a way for women to address their fears and anxieties in a safe way.

What if we were to view each environment where birth takes place as one that is a 'sacred space' to be respected and treated with awe? Would we change the trappings within the space, make it more comfortable and comforting? Would we walk softly, speak respectfully and calmly, and encourage others to do the same? Would we slow down? Would we reconsider the ability for people to enter the space without knocking and being invited in?

What if midwives were truly able to 'be' there and 'hold the space', enabling a woman to feel safe to go into her 'zone' during labour. What if midwives and medical staff were able to support partners to support the women better? What would it be like if midwives and doctors could freely speak about spirituality and childbirth without fear of being ridiculed?

What if we were to recognise the spiritual nature of the unborn baby as well? Would we start to question some of the actions we take or offer through pregnancy, labour and beyond? Would it help us to respect more deeply the strength of the mother-baby dyad and invest more in nurturing this relationship from conception, or even pre-conception, to support the wellbeing of the mother, and therefore the growing unborn?

What if we were able to have all the time possible to listen to women during the childbirth continuum and help them to make the right decisions for their situation and for their baby or to alleviate their fear and anxieties? Would this enable us to find out where they gain their strength and the rich meanings they hold onto from the everyday?

We hope this collection of thought-provoking diverse chapters raises conscious awareness about spirituality and childbirth. The lived reality of childbirth as highlighted repeatedly in these pages challenges the assumption that the phenomenon of childbirth is purely secular. Perhaps you are now able to resonate with the notion that 'there is something going on at birth', and agree that something more than a purely secular lens is required to appreciate the mystery of childbirth? We need a changing story of childbirth that attunes spirituality, tactful practice, sensitivity, compassion and a new way of connectedness transcending differences. The meaning of childbirth to professionals and society as a whole requires our combined thinking lest something of importance is lost. The voices in this book will encourage engagement with this changing story about childbirth; a story that is of celebration of a shared natality not merely a story about mortality and morbidity avoidance.

We believe there are wider concerns that are evolving over time that we are unable to ignore – that of sustainability of our planet and of humanity. How we attune to childbirth in our collective and individual lives is fundamental to our continuance as a meaning-making species that thrives on connectedness. The continuation of our species requires focus on interconnectedness with all things including the environment and our relationship to the Earth. For a sustainable future we need to honour, shelter and nurture how life begets life. How we attend and attune to childbirth and our Earth is crucial for our survival. If these assertions are correct then the implications in *Spirituality and Childbirth: Meaning and Care at the Start of Life* need our full attention through education, research, policy and practice lest we lose something of existential significance and forget that it ever existed. That would be a travesty. Childbirth is a gift in our individual and collective, personal and professional lives often bringing joy and possibilities for new tomorrows; let us take care and honour this precious gift.

INDEX

Taylor & Francis eBooks

Helping you to choose the right eBooks for your Library

Add Routledge titles to your library's digital collection today. Taylor and Francis ebooks contains over 50,000 titles in the Humanities, Social Sciences, Behavioural Sciences, Built Environment and Law.

Choose from a range of subject packages or create your own!

Benefits for you

>> Free MARC records
>> COUNTER-compliant usage statistics
>> Flexible purchase and pricing options
>> All titles DRM-free.

Benefits for your user

>> Off-site, anytime access via Athens or referring URL
>> Print or copy pages or chapters
>> Full content search
>> Bookmark, highlight and annotate text
>> Access to thousands of pages of quality research at the click of a button.

REQUEST YOUR **FREE** INSTITUTIONAL TRIAL TODAY

Free Trials Available
We offer free trials to qualifying academic, corporate and government customers.

eCollections – Choose from over 30 subject eCollections, including:

Archaeology	Language Learning
Architecture	Law
Asian Studies	Literature
Business & Management	Media & Communication
Classical Studies	Middle East Studies
Construction	Music
Creative & Media Arts	Philosophy
Criminology & Criminal Justice	Planning
Economics	Politics
Education	Psychology & Mental Health
Energy	Religion
Engineering	Security
English Language & Linguistics	Social Work
Environment & Sustainability	Sociology
Geography	Sport
Health Studies	Theatre & Performance
History	Tourism, Hospitality & Events

For more information, pricing enquiries or to order a free trial, please contact your local sales team: www.tandfebooks.com/page/sales